The Invisible Stalker

I0117997

Patricia Reid

chipmunkapublishing
the mental health publisher

Patricia Reid

Published by
Chipmunkapublishing
PO Box 6872
Brentwood
Essex CM13 1ZT
United Kingdom

http://www.chipmunkapublishing.com

Chipmunkapublishing gratefully acknowledge the support of Arts Council England.

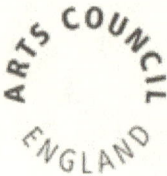

ARTS COUNCIL ENGLAND

The Invisible Stalker

Acknowledgements

I am here to tell the tale because of a few good people. That is a fact. I want to thank them for their undying support in my toughest times, and not giving up on me or judging me because I have a mental illness.
 They are all very important to me.

They are Aaron Hart who saved my life this last time; Kirsty Pleace who saved my life the time before; The Brewer mob which are: Leonie, Grant, (who had to come a very long way around the harbour in the middle of the night a few times to get me when I was near the edge of reason. Along with Nichola, Sam and Leah, the kids, who give the best hugs on the planet. (thanks for your bed Sam as you had to sleep on the sofa when I was brought to your house by your parents); Penny and Graham for being the most funny and loving people; Natalie Jane, my gentle, beautiful daughter-in-law and not least of all, my two son's Luke and Justin Reid who without missing a beat, give me mountains of love, affection and unwaivering support. They are my rock and they have given me so much to hold onto and more. I love you, I am honoured to be your mother.

And Ruth Ross, my enduring, tireless psychologist who gave me the tools to fight and see another day, and another, and another. My family thanks you for giving me back the power to fight this mental illness. I am still here.

Patricia Reid

The Invisible Stalker

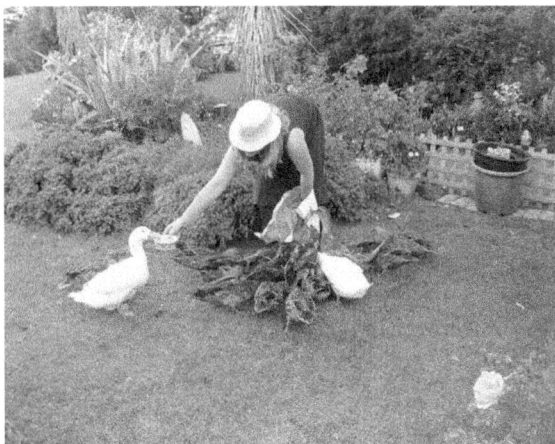

Patricia Reid

CHAPTER ONE

This picture shows me feeding my ducks. I am someone who looks to be content. It is amazing what we see as reality, is far far from the truth. On the day this picture was taken, I overdosed with a huge concoxion of drugs with the intentions and determination of taking my own life. How can anyone possibly know beforehand that someone they hold dear is about to commit suicide? Personally I think that is very hard to do. I am not talking about the people who cry out for help, yes, they let you know how they feel, and may indeed feel suicidal, and should be taken seriously. But the people who do follow through and commit suicide, they generally do this without any fuss or attention drawn to themselves. Quietly.

I was feeling OK when I got up that morning. Infact I can generally tell when I first wake up what my day is going to be like and if I will have a battle on my hands with depression or, getting through the day with a semblance of contentment which is like winning the lottery. I dragged myself out of bed that morning, nearly standing on Black Puss, my 10 year old back cat. . (yeah, original name for a black cat. The imagination was not flowing with cat names when we got him and his sister, who is gray and is called Gray Puss).Anyway, he was prancing around my feet in his eagerness to get my attention to the most urgent message of his life and that was he's hungry and wanted his breakfast NOW! If you have a cat, you can appreciate how demanding they can be. So to give me some breathing space and also to stop the little buggers from bothering me, first things first in the Reid household and that is feed the cats. There is no peace until that job is done. The cats both make it their business to do this ritualistic dance around my feet from the moment my feet touch the floor in my bedroom, until I get the food out of the fridge for them and into their bowls. Then, and only then, do they stop hassling me and eat their breakfast. (Generally I don't see them until the evening when they come home and start demanding a warm lap to curl up on for the evening). Only then can I go up and have my shower and get myself ready for the day ahead.

I like to go outside first thing in the morning to focus and remind myself of my surroundings and to take in the beauty of the harbor view with the sun just peeking out over the horizon. The red-and-black sunrise slowly changes to one of gold and red, which also looks magnificent. It is too easy to lose sight of this beauty as I drown in my head. I focus on the trees and the harbor and really look at them. This is an exercise I have to do to make sure I am in the here and now and to keep the emotions upbeat and under tight control. It is too easy to rush off somewhere and not notice the lovely garden you plant, or the changing colors of the trees, which in themselves can be quite spectacular. If I don't do this, in its place, all I can visualize is more threat, destruction and cruelty in the world we live in. This makes me anxious. And when I get anxious it escalates into catastrophe so when I go outside to see the beauty all around me, I feel better about the day ahead.

 Sadly, I have reached this place in my life where even small hiccups in my day can seem humongous and overwhelming. It is as if there is a switch in my brain that flicks to "panic mode". Then there is a sense of complete panic and I suddenly don't know what I am supposed to do, what my role is in life, where I fit in, in the scheme of things. My mind goes blank. It is a very isolating place to find myself in. This makes me want to run away from myself, die, anything to get away from these feelings. I really have to try and focus to combat this on a daily basis.

I need to have some semblance of order in my day otherwise I risk spinning out into the grip of helplessness and despair. I have found that I can barely function to the same capacity I once did.

Recently when I was visiting my son in his office, and bemoaned my life to him, telling him I feel like a total failure, he takes me seriously because of my mental illness. He knew these feelings are a precursor to me going downhill. Knowing this I had to seek out my son for my wellbeing.

In his usual fashion, Luke listened to me, then pulled out of his bag of knowledge a reminder of what I have done with my life. He decided we should make up my resume. With me putting things into perspective this way helped. Yes I was surprised at what I have achieved in my life. The variety of jobs and skill levels amazed me. For instance, when I look back on career choices I made, it is hard to believe now that I had a high stress job in the bank and did it with ease. I could talk investments or borrowing with the customer with confidence. But now, I couldn't even talk to people without panicking and feeling inferior. I used to be an ambulance officer where you had to have your wits about you and know your stuff. That job was a high stress job also with having to consider your safety, the safety of your patient and most importantly making sure your actions were the right actions and procedures to keep your patient calm and from declining and dying if possible. I could do this. I could do this with ease and compassion. Now I am not sure I could put a band aide on a cut finger. My confidence and self esteem has gone down the plug hole. I feel as though I have burnt myself out.

So again, with infinite patience, my son reminded me of

a recent trip I took to the outback of Australia. Oh yes, do I remember this trip very well.

I felt it was necessary for me to face myself and my demons. I also felt it necessary to write about suicide, depression and how terrible it was. Also I was fed up with being anxious all the time and I needed to be on my own and what better place than in the middle of the Australian outback. Of course, I didn't tell my boys my motive for going on this trip. I didn't want them to worry, or worse, stop me going. I told them I wanted an adventure and after a lot of persuasion, I was on my way. So off I went to Australia with my dogs. I bought a campervan when I got there as this was going to be my home and transport for the next while. I didn't' know how long I was going for, but was determined to push my boundaries and get out of my comfort zone. In a way it was like I wanted to go and fight for me and my survival. I honestly didn't know if I was going to live or die there. I had to do this for me. I did push my boundaries. I did get out of my comfort zone and I did survive even in adversity.

One of the incidents Luke reminded me of was when I was in the desert and was days away from anywhere. My campervan got stuck in the sand. I had no phone signal and no one knew where I was. I usually drove where the fancy took me. If a dirt road looked interesting, well I would go down it and see where it went to. I had no "plan" like any sensible tourist. I wanted to be lost. I didn't want to know where I was going. I just drove. Maybe I was trying to drive away from my demons, but I just drove until I got tired then set up camp. I liked it this way. Anyway, I was on my own. Well, I had my two small dogs with me on this journey and that was comforting.

The Invisible Stalker

There was dust everywhere. You cannot keep it down. It is in your mouth, up your nose, ears, hair, clothes and in the food. This area we were in (roughly east a couple of days of carnarvon which is on the west coast somewhere if I remember rightly) is windy so there is always a dust storm. The dogs didn't seem to care, they rolled in the sand and of course found any dead things within sniffing distance, so enjoyed themselves regardless. We were stuck in the sand for two days. I tried different ways to get out of the sand but as I tried, so the van just dug deeper and even further until the (axle) was touching the ground. I realised there was more thinking needed and I wish I could call up McGivor with his penknife and tape, but he probably wasn't home! damb.

The dogs tried to help me dig out the tires but I was worried they would get buried too so wouldn't let them near the van. Ewok, my Shisu whined allot and Muscha, my Pomeranian looked at him in bewilderment and just sat there. So, with a dust pan, I dug down, put dried bracken under they tyres, (nothing else around), but this did not work. I was in the middle of nowhere and with no phone reception, no main roads near by and defiantly no traffic. I had to look upon this as a Girl Scout challenge. The first and most important job I figured was to get myself a diet coke from the fridge. (it didn't help the situation much, but it tasted good as it was very hot and dry out there).

Talking away to my dogs, I explained the next action plan which was I needed to go pee. I went in the potty, and then, like an ingenious thought striking me, (see, it was the coke) I tipped the pee out onto the sand by the tires, to make the sand more viscous and hoped it would help grip. The sand was fine and dry and kept caving in every time I tried to dig it out to put bracken there.

Then I had another ingenious thought, eat. So I got some chocolate out the fridge, mmmmm, nothing like cold chocolate and coke to help you through a challenge. Well nothing was working so far after hours trying to dig my way out. I had to think of drastic measures as I was running out of water and food. I knew this was it. It was the last ditch attempt to get myself out of this mess because no one was going to come and rescue me. No one knew where I was and I was off the beaten track which didn't help. I had to look at my resources. I had water I could use to wet the area to stop the sand caving in all the time, but then I knew that would be it. If it didn't work I would be stuffed. To have no water with you in the desert is not a good thing. It was a gamble but there was nothing else I could think of. I needed to make the sand wet to stop it moving all the time which would give me a chance to get out. I also took my bed to pieces (I made it with bits of wood) and shoved the wood under the van and put the car jack there to prop up the van as much as I could.

Then I would fill in the hole with sand and repeat this until the tyres were nearly level with the ground. Then using the last of the the water to wet the area and towels, I shoved this under the tyres. This was it, I had nothing else. I was all out of ideas by this time and if this didn't work, well. After praying with my pooches, I got back into the van for the hundredth time, turned the key and looked at my dogs thinking this may be the place where we all perish if this doesn't work. I slowly put my foot down on the excellerator, expecting nothing but spinning tyres again. But the van moved. I couldn't believe it. It worked. The van drove out of the hole with the makeshift flooring I put under the tyres. I was back onto firm ground again. I was whooping and yelling and was really pleased with myself as I had saved us from catastrophe, and the ironic thing was if we did die out there, the boys may think it was suicide when infact it wasn't. The dogs thought this was too much excitement for one day and curled up on the front seat and went to sleep as I drove us to civilization with a smirky grin and feeling very pleased with myself for getting us out of that bad situation.

I eventually got to a town (without any further mishaps) and found a cool internet café and went in with two very tired dogs, which fell asleep under the table at my feet. (It was very hot in the dessert) I had no bed to speak of, but hay, who cares, the bits of wood broke with the weight of the van). The situation was almost comical.
I looked like a dirty dusty tramp just come to town after lying in the hot sand for two days digging.

Oh yes, before we went to the desert, we were near Perth, just got there, and set up camp in the woods. Ewok, my shisu came rushing back to the camper (I was working on this book) and he drove his face into the bed and was going crazy. I thought this strange behaviour so I had a look and realized his muzzle was swelling up. I immediately thought spider, snakes, so rushed outside and saw what it was, I didn't see it before I set up camp but there was lots of bee hives around the side of some bushes. Ewok had obviously stuck his nose in where he shouldn't have, and got stung by a few angry bees. Not sure how many stings, so I stood there thinking about this and wondering about where to get some antihistamine, then suddenly Muscha yelped. I assumed he got stung too, but he immediately acted very strange. He stood there for a moment, then vomited and then had a seizure and went unconscious. I immediately thought of a snake. Especially as his reaction was so fast and acute.

I couldn't believe that within two minutes of each other,

Ewok and Muscha where in trouble and I needed a vet urgently. What a coincidence. I didn't know I could move so fast. I had to do CPR on Muscha as he had stopped breathing and was limp. I was desperately trying to hold it together and in between this was shoving stuff in the van while massaging Muscha little chest. Thanks to my GPS I could find a vet within a short time. I think I broke the sound barrier in my haste to get to the vets, driving with one hand on the wheel and massaging Muscha's chest with the other. I looked over at Ewok and his mouth was getting huge and he was looking at me so pathetically as only they can do. (I was imagining him going into anaphylactic shock from the swelling which was freaking me out).

I was very worried and extremely stressed. I got to the vets very quickly thanks to the GPS (my son Luke bought it for me for my travels around Australia and that was the best gift I ever have).
I ran into the vets with my poor dogs and the vet saw them straight away. Muscha was bitten by either a spider or a particular ant that is bad news like a fire ant or a green ant, but not a snake. The vet said he would be dead if he was bitten by a snake being such a small dog.

The dogs both had injections to stop the effects of their encounters with the creepy crawlies. What a relief. I was so pathetically grateful they were going to be ok. We celebrated by me having greasy fish and chips. The dogs didn't want to eat for the rest of the day, but I got them some fresh chicken the next day which they loved.

When we got back to a town we stayed at a lovely camping ground which allows dogs! It had all these lovely ducks, peacocks, geese and birds there, as there is a big pond area where they stay. But due to my

The Invisible Stalker

pooches being over friendly with the aquatic life, I am not sure we will be invited back because the first thing Ewok did while I was setting up camp, was, yeah, chase the ducks and what a ruckus they made as they scampered back to the pond for safety, with feathers flying and kicking up the dust on the path. So I quickly got his lead from the van to tie him up so he couldn't'[t get into any more mischief but as soon as I turned around he was gone again, chasing the (turkeys I think) and I could hear them all squawking as they ran for their lives. I of course, ran after him again, feeling like an inadequate mother but trying not to show it and with an authoritive sounding voice, I yelled for him to stop, heel, come as he continued in his persuit and proceeded to ignore me, running after the poor birds. The birds couldn't fly which I'm sure delighted Ewok as he gave a good chase. He stopped chasing them when HE decided to, not his mistress who was threatening all kinds of gruesome things to him when I caught him. He had the nerve to look very happy as he trotted back to me, panting away and wagging his tail... I had to take a picture of his comical face.

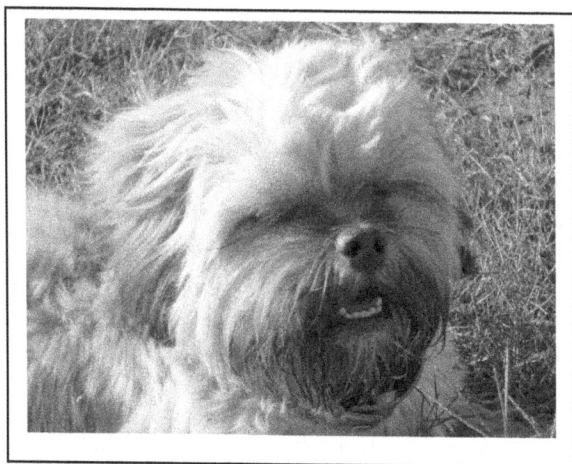

This was 5 minutes into our stay at this lovely place. I expected the man to come down and kick us out, but no one came thank goodness. I put him on a long lead and tied it to a tree thinking he couldn't get into anymore trouble while I continued to set up camp and do lunch.

By the time I had finished, about15 minutes, I got suspicious as Ewok was quiet....he usually harasses me to play or barks at every moving thing he sees, so I thought I'd better check out what he was up to or if he had escaped and was munching on a turkey leg or something..but no, when I found him at the end of the long lead, he had decided to explore the ravine which I didn't know was there, as there are lots of bushes hiding it.

What I found was this mud covered dog with his head in a hole he was digging out...but it was all silt and he was half in the water while he was doing this. He looked up and his face was all black with a pink tongue poking out. He looked very funny. Seeing him in this state I just gave up and just left him digging down to whatever juicy bones he thinks was down there.

When I had finished setting up camp, my next job was to get Ewok cleaned up before he was allowed back in the campervan. Of course dogs are not allowed in the showers so wondered what to do to get all that mud off him, and by this time he was covered, except for a small patch on his back, he missed that. I guess he couldn't get into the hole enough to completely cover himself. I thought about it, and wondered how I was going to get him cleaned up. Of course he wanted to jump all over me, making me muddy too. I guess he wanted to show me how mud is so cooling, so try some.

So, I picked him up, and marched him off to the pond and threw him in. Sorted!. But I had forgotten about the geese who were harassed so shortly beforehand and were not amused that the little terror was back and in their pond, I can tell you. I could see the geese making a beeline for us...they were in the middle of the pond at this time. I had just enough time to throw Ewok in the pond again to get the last of the mud off him before the geese got to us. I got most of the mud off him anyway so that was good, but the main goose got to the shore near us, hissing and carrying on as we backed off away from their pond. I was ok about letting the goose peck Ewok (not too hurt him as such but to let him know birds can retaliate, so stop chasing them.) The goose started to chase Ewok and he quickly realised the goose wanted to get him so ran behind my legs for me to protect him, great. So there was the goose in front of my legs hissing away and Ewok behind me expecting me to come to his rescue. The goose could not get to him so I'm sure out of pure frustration, took it out on me and decided to peck at my legs and shoes. I took photos as we were backing away from it, but it followed and was able to peck Ewok eventually. He let out a loud yelp, even though I am sure the goose never really hurt him, just his pride, but we got away.

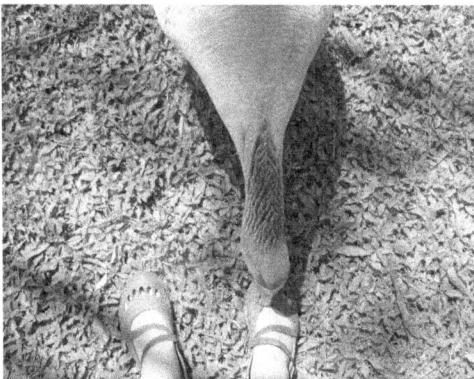

Now when we walk past the pond, Ewok gives the fowl a wide birth!!)

Now all this, with the recent desert thing was stressful but I was fine. There was no depression to be seen in all this time. It crept up on me a few months later. If given a choice, I would rather face a pride of lions and take my chances than this mind controlling depression any day. I control it the best way I can with the aide of medication and various other tools like relaxation therapy and exercise, I generally manage OK and get through, but some days are tougher than others, like the day I was feeding my ducks.

This day was just another ordinary day; no dramas. I was functioning fine and going about my business as normal at home in wonderful Dunedin. Dunedin is where the Royal Albatross have lived for many a secure year thanks to the help of DOC (Department of Conservation along with a few dedicated volunteers), on the Otago peninsula.

Outwardly, I look the typically content middle-aged woman who seams to have everything, especially the most precious of all: my two sons. They are twenty-nine and twenty-seven, respectively. I am happy to say we are very close as a family. Their father lives in the USA mostly but makes time to see them, which is good. Yes, I have no complaints, except this one thing that has dogged my life. Depression.

I am not a clinician of any kind. I do not have any qualifications in the mental-health sector, but what I do have is unwanted experience of depression and of attempting suicide by means that should have done the job effectively. By giving you first hand information into how someone like myself who has a good life, can do

The Invisible Stalker

this, it may help you understand the devastating effects depression can have on someone like your loved ones too. If you have lost someone to suicide you may be searching for answers. I do not have the answers to your pain; I only have my experience to share with you. And by that, it may help you understand a little why someone could possibly do such a thing to themselves and leave behind devastation and confusion. I will describe the depth I had to reach before I contemplated suicide.

The people who took their lives cannot come back and tell you how they felt prior to exiting this life or why they did it — how they felt even. But if they could, I would bet a bottom dollar that they would tell you they were not in their right minds at the time, figuratively speaking.

When I am deeply depressed, I write. In a way it is like a lifeline for me to write how I feel at that moment. It is the only thing I can do when I am in the black hole. I write as if my life depends on it. Usually it is about how I am feeling at that moment. Imagine being very, very drunk and then writing how you feel at that moment. The concentration is acute as you have to make the brain perform a task when all it really wants to do is black out. The handwriting change, as it is hard to write when the head is not "with it," so my writing looks very childish, but has the essence of how I felt while in the black hole. Sometimes the writing is illegible, but can be deciphered. I know I have this burning need to explain to my sons why I am killing myself. So I write my way through the experience as I wait to die. I am being consumed by mental torture and it is blinding. You cannot think straight or logically, even though you may think your thinking through things logically, but your not. The mind can be very deceptive and give all the wrong messages even if it is detrimental to your wellbeing.

This is what this book is really about. If you have lost someone to suicide, then this may be worth reading. They had their reasons why they died, yes, but logic no. that goes out the window with sanity. But the emotional pain — the whole barrel of emotions that we experience — is there; one hundred fold, crushing us. We are then lost in the depression until it lifts again to free us for a time, or kill's us. This is like a silent stalker; depression.

This subject is important to me because I think there is little real understanding about suicide. This is my story of doing just that: committing suicide. The fact that I failed is irrelevant; for all intents and purposes, I committed an act that should have killed me.

And so this book, I hope, will give you some insight as to my last moments of how I felt before the act itself — taking the drugs — and then waiting to be released. The defining moment, if you like, of what my mind is telling me.

I myself was incapable of thinking rationally at the time prior to my self-destruction. So it may help you to know that the person you lost, was for a while, lost to reality for that time. I was lost too. I never gave my beautiful sons a thought other than practical stuff, because I became devoid of emotions. However, I did survive where others did not. I am eternally grateful that I did not hurt my boys. In a way the people who did succeed, I want to say that they didn't do it consciously to hurt anyone they loved. They were lost and couldn't find their way back in time.

This book is for their loved ones who have to continue life's journey without them. I could have died also and then there would have been no one to explain to my sons in a empathic way that I had a mental illness and this was the reason their mum left them this way... and certainly not because she did not love them because she did, with all her heart.

CHAPTER TWO

My garden has many ducks; predominately mallards, but they have their own unique beauty. A few of them have made it their permanent home all year round, so I have gotten to know them better and has enabled me to distinguish which is which and who is who. They have personalities — yeah, really! I can imagine you thinking, she is nuts, of course they don't, they are only ducks for goodness sake! However, they do and duck nuts can back me up on that!

For instance, one of the mallards (a female) who have been here for a few years now, is Miss Quackless. She does not have a quack, or a voice for a better word.
She is always the first duck to waddle up to me (so I think she is the bravest of them all) and demands food by quacking but without a sound. I immediately get her wheat, letting her know I heard her loud and clear, metaphorically speaking. She is a bossy thing because if I am not quick smart, she pecks my toes. (No, it doesn't hurt at all; it is more a gesture to hurry me up!) I do not know what happened for her to lose her voice but she certainly makes herself understood.

She is also a survivor. One day she turned up on my driveway, and I immediately knew there was something wrong because she just sat there. She never just sits there. She is demanding when she comes in from the harbor as she waddles up to me with that funny gait they have and demand food soundlessly. (Silence can be deafening!) All the ducks tend to follow me around when there is the hope of extra food going spare and they do not settle down until I either go into the house or feed them. Anyway, Miss Quackless was sitting on the driveway this particular morning instead of following me around with the rest of ducks.

I took a couple of steps towards her and still she did not get up, which is not normal. I figured there must be something wrong with her, and being a die-hard animal lover that I am, I became concerned. So trying to make myself unthreatening (I never approach the ducks, I let them come to me), I crept up to her very slowly (she is still wild and her survival skills wanted to kick in and flee the blobby old girl with the silly straw hat, but she couldn't.)

She tried to stand but there was something wrong with her leg, so she tried to move out of my reach by using her wings to maneuver her further down the path, which, of course, just made me feel awful for her plight. But I had to get hold of her, so feeling bad — knowing I would probably frighten her half to death — I just had to take the plunge and pounce on her; well not pounce as in the image of flattening her with my hefty weight. I moved fast enough to grab her before she moved and hurt herself even more. She was not happy about being handled by a gross, featherless giant and tried to flap her wings in protest. I held her wings down very gently but she was strong, so I had to apply a little more pressure to control her flapping and murmured the usual crap we think is reassuring to our pets that are in distress. The other ducks also showed a vote of extreme displeasure by taking off in a swarm of flying feathers, pooping and quacking very loudly. There are roughly thirty-something ducks at any one time in my garden, so they can make quite a din when they are alarmed. That is how I know I have visitors — the ducks warn me. Great alarm system!

When she stopped trying to get away and settled down, I examined her legs and found one of the knee joints (if that is what it is called) was swollen quite badly, hence the reason she could not walk. I felt a little relieved that it was nothing more serious like a broken leg, which would mean a visit to the vet's office. This does not bear thinking about. In addition, my boys would really think I had lost my marbles at last!

As it is, my sons love ducks for different reasons; they eat them and pay approximately thirty dollars for a small duck at the butcher. So for me to take a wild duck to the vet and pay a huge amount of money to save its life is beyond their comprehension. (And most duck hunters, I imagine!).

I took the duck into the house and did what every doting mother would do: I got her some nice soggy bread with wheat thrown in for good measure and gave it to her.
She looked at me straight in the eyes as if trying to figure out what my agenda was — like fattening her up for the pot, for instance! I can't imagine why wild ducks don't trust us!

But hunger got the better of her and I like to think she decided I was not going to eat her after all and to just go with it, thus she ate the soggy bread goop as if she had not eaten in months.

I like to think that was when she decided to trust me. She allowed me to care for her until her leg healed to the point that she could limp around without too much discomfort. She never makes a sound and just does the actions as if she is quacking — and boy can she be a nag when she wants to!

The ducks nest in the bushes by the pond and have their offspring, despite the family cats, of which I have two. This is Miss Quackless with her brood; she is a good mother and is the most successful of the ducks in raising most of her ducklings to adulthood.

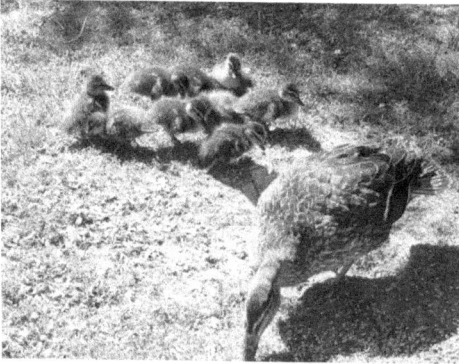

As in the human species, there are some badass mother#%@*@ out there too! This morning when I walked through the hallway to the kitchen, I happened to glance outside the front window to get a glimpse of the ducks and to also see if there are any more ducklings on the lawn as it was the season for new arrivals of the cute fluffy things; seeing them always gives me a lift.

To my horror, what I did see was one of the mother ducks throwing a duckling up in the air and then letting it fall to the ground, landing on its back. Then this duck viciously pecked the duckling's soft belly a couple of times, showing not an ounce of mercy and then grabbing it by its soft belly and throwing the poor thing into the air again and landing on the ground — it would repeatedly carry out this awful behavior.

It was so bazaar I could not quite grasp the situation. I stood there, mouth open, unable to do anything but just stare in horror, which seemed like hours but was really only a second or two, I expect. (If Stephan King studied the duck society, he could get some good ideas for a horror story that would chill the most ardent, hardhearted fans.)

I noticed in the millisecond of taking in this horror show that the mother duck had two small ducklings of her own. This duckling was trying to join a family, as, for whatever reason, it obviously had none of its own. It was desperately trying to attach itself to this family of ducks, even though the mother was attacking it, with only one aim in mind — to kill it. It was heart wrenching to see this happening to the poor thing. It was only a few days old and scared. (The same size as the ones in the picture). It had no mother duck to care for it. In a pitiful attempt at self-preservation, it had tried to get up and run into the hedge to hide from its attacker.

I felt quite sick inside to think even these lovely friends of mine, as that is what they are to me, could be brutal to each other. Then this triggered me thinking of all the cruelty in the world. Humans killing their babies, animals do the same, like the lion killing another lion's cub so it could procreate with the lioness. I felt very angry at this world of destruction, then so deflated knowing there is nothing that can be done about it. The world is what it is, I know, but it doesn't make me feel any better about it.

I have been feeding the ducks for the last six years and there has always be an abundance of food to go around, yet the survival instincts had caused her to behave in this barbaric way. Kill or be killed seems to be the motto for animals on this planet. I love the Animal Channel with the amazing documentaries of wildlife, but even then I have to turn away when the wild animals hunt for dinner and start the chase of some poor gazelle or zebra that it can take down. I do find it hard to watch. Plus due to my lack of a tough outer shell, I get overly sensitive to things around me and can easily get down about it.

There is not enough of a tolerance level for me from being OK to being very depressed. I wish I had some gray areas, as this is the cushion you need to stop falling down the black hole to despair.

Anyway, horror of all horrors, the poor thing sees this giant of a creature come shooting out of the house towards it, shouting loudly. At that moment, the mother duck gave one last peck of the duckling before she decided it was time to push off and protect her own offspring. She scooted away with them to the relative safety of the pond, away from this charging mad woman.

So in this moment of reprieve from the brutal bill bashing it received, the little duckling managed to struggle up on such little wobbly legs and by sheer terror, it ran as fast as it could to hide under the thick carpet of rose bushes just as I got there. The poor little thing was able to escape this further horror of a giant in its very short life.

When after trying to reach it under very prickly bush and being scratched by the thorns in the process, I had to admit defeat — I could not reach the duckling. My attempts to get it just added to the poor thing's fear, so I went back inside the house and hoped that the little thing found its own mother soon, but in the meantime I would keep an eye out for it if possible. Meanwhile, I would work on not getting anxious about it. This sort of thing can make me think about what lives on this planet and how brutal it all seems. I have to work hard not to think, switching it off if possible, which you know is not an easy thing to do!

After about ten minutes of glancing out of the window, I saw the ducks had come back to the front lawn. Then I noticed the little orphan duckling slowly come out from under the rose bushes but it did not venture any further and stayed near the bushes as if it was nervous about coming out into the open. I could see it looking around at all the ducks as if it was looking for its own mother. It looked so forlorn; it made my heart ache for it. (At that moment, I could relate to its being out of the fold, unprotected and alone. I grew up feeling like this from early childhood.)

Ducks were walking around and some were preening themselves. The little duckling must have felt reassured that it was not going to be attacked, so it came out onto the lawn, but watching the ducks as it did, it skirted around the edge of the shrubbery to avoid any ducks that came its way. I decided to watch and wait to see what happened; hoping very much that it would find its mother, or possibly its mother would find its offspring.

The little thing must have felt more confident because nothing bad had happened so far, so it ventured out further away from the rose bushes. But for some unfathomable reason, it had another go at bonding with the same duck that had attacked it not so long ago. (I know this because this particular duck had only two offspring, where the other ducks had six or more.)

I was surprised to find the gorgeous, fluffy ducklings of each family chasing away other impostors that would try to muscle in on its family group! They all look the same, but they all know who their siblings are and who are not!

Well, this mother duck spotted it and again and attacked the poor thing vigorously. I dashed outside to rescue the duckling from the attack, but when I got to it, it did not run away as it had done previously.

I thought the duckling was dead when I reached it because it was lying on its back not moving, just lying there very still. I felt terrible for it and angry at the ducks for their brutality and God for creating a world full of such brutality. Never mind free will, this duckling had no free will. Do I get pecked to death or don't I?

I am still trying to understand why terrible things happen. If this is God's creation, what sort of God is it to create such a brutal way to survive?

I picked it up thinking it was dead, and then realized it was still alive, but looked dead, as it was limp and lifeless in the palm of my hand. It was as if the duckling was in shock. Then it moved slightly to my relief and looked right at me with those little dark eyes while lying on its back in my hands, as if to say, oh no, this featherless giant is going to eat me now.

My heart hurt so badly for that poor duckling, lying there in my hand, so fragile, like a newborn baby. It reminded me of the picture I painted for myself, symbolically showing me as a baby being protected by someone who cared. The picture I am referring to is at the end of the book. Especially when I was at school, I seemed to be always in trouble with the teachers. (I'm sure it had nothing to do with me being a smelly dirty kid who never saw a hair brush or tooth brush for that matter. Oh and the nits and fleas I suppose! I was blissfully unaware of my appearance, being a child of course and not understanding adults had an aversion to dirty kids (other peoples of course). So being used to being yelled at often, I imagine being in the kind hand of God, being protected from the outside world which seemed horrible at times. In fact, if you can wear out a mental picture by constant use, it would be in crumbly pieces by now.

Now I am an adult, I am aware of the fact that adults can be abrasive and have little understanding or tolerance towards children's feelings. If anything, children feel things more acutely of what is going on around them but are dismissed because adults assume they know nothing or feel nothing of any relevance. Children learn from adults and they want to be doing the right thing, whatever that is. All for approval and importantly love. Which some children just don't get. They are the unfortunate ones with a shaky journey ahead of them. They can live in a castle or a shack but If they grow up without the love they need to survive this life, it becomes that much tougher a journey. I believe every single one of us, unless you are made of stone, craves to be loved. Period. It moulds you. It makes you. It breaks you. It is necessary. Even though it is a duckling of no significant to the world in general, it needs the love of its mother to nurture it and help it survive in this world of ours. Or a miracle and they don't come around too often.

Well here we are again, the duckling is so reliant on its parent for survival, but it has no protection, no mother duck to protect it. so vulnerable to attack and could not defend itself. I wanted to find the "creator" and peck him or her to death for allowing such pain and suffering in the world. You have to be pretty tough to live in this world because we are exposed to so much negativity and violence on TV or newspapers or schools or movies. Even the kids now-a-days are playing computer games where they blow things up or shoot someone. They hypothetically become a crack shots before they go to school! Hmmm how do we protect our kids from such things? You don't seem to see kids out on the streets playing anymore, the parks are deserted now apart from a parent with a young child or two. You don't see teenagers having fun in parks. It seams to have gone, along with the flower power days. The kids are somewhere more isolated now like in their bedroom playing on the computer, having access to all sorts of unmentionable horrors that can be accessed via the internet. Some parents who are not savvy with the internet will have no idea just what cam be obtained and downloaded onto little johnnies computer. Why can't they just go outside and have a water fight with their friends instead? Or climb a tree or two. Cricket and football was very common to see on the streets or on waste land, but not now. I remember we had so much fun with other kids in the streets. We played hide and seek (yep, even the bigger kids like the challenge of not being found till last). And marbles was very popular with the kids. Kids that had marbles always had a "favourite" marble. But in the game, they had the risk of losing the favourite marble in a game. They would try to win it back and if they did would feel like the king of the street. But if they didn't they went home with a determination stronger than Winston Churchill's wanting to win the war, and was hell bent on getting their favourite marble back the next game they played with their opponent.

If you couldn't afford marbles as some kids couldn't, it didn't matter, there was a game of conkers and conkers was free. But you still had your favourite, shinny concer that stayed intact and become the champion concer of the street. To play conkers, you had to find the biggest, best concer possible in the fields. They you would get a nail and or something sharp and pierce a hole through the middle of the conker and thread a string through it and tie a knot at the end, so that the string did not come back through. This then becomes your tool for a great game of conkers. You have to knock the other opponent's conker until it breaks up and comes off the string. If yours is still intact, you are the winner, with a prize conker!! It was serious stuff and not a drop of blood was spilt! We then went home with our gains, determination for another day and pride in our hearts. And of course, starving.

I feel things too deeply, which sometimes overwhelm me, like this incident with the duckling. I just want to yell, scream, and bash something, anything for the injustices in the world and where we are going as a race. One thing I can say about religion, you would be too scared to do anything wrong incase you got struck down by God or lightening or something just as scary. So we behaved generally. But there is not the same trust for religions now-a-days as there is so much conflict associated with them.

I feel ashamed of being human because all I can see is bad outweighing good, but I am sure this is not the case really — right? I have to focus on the good to keep from going into despair. I feel I cannot take any more emotional beatings. But I seam to and survive them. And now I can feel all the negative things regarding this world starting to crowd my mind and makes me want to get off the planet.

I looked down at the little guy and I have to be focused and stop negative thinking, so pulling myself together, I wanted this little guy to have a chance to live, against the odds. Being it is so young, a day or two but no more, I was not sure if it got any internal damage, let alone shock, but I had to try. I was giving the Gods the fingers and was going to do everything in my power to help it survive. I would look after it myself. I put it down my t-shirt to keep it warm and see if it would recover a little more first. It took about half an hour for it to start moving and squeaking, which made me feel such relief.

The Invisible Stalker

With hope in my heart, I got to it and made the specialty of the day: duckling cuisine. Well, actually, it is a mushy, smelly mess that ducks seem to love called cat biscuit soup! I mix cat biscuits and hot water to make it all mushy for little beaks. It has a good sauce of nutrients, if it is to have a chance to recover.

I have raised ducklings a few times in the past, (strays) mainly piiking ducks, as they do not make the best parents so am amazed they are not extinct now! The cutest duckling I raised was a paradise duck (female). I called her Ducky...yeah, so original. She was found alone in some woods wandering about and looking very lost. She was only a day or two old, so a friend rescued her and brought her to me to raise. She is happy raising her own family now. She comes back every year and nests in the paddock next door.

I make sure I remember all the good things around me because if I do not, it is as if I have a hole in my head and bad memories start to take over. Thus, it is important for me to focus on the good things every day. Like the success stories of life. One success story is that every morning I come downstairs and if there is not a dead duckling on the hall floor, kindly deposited by black puss, then that is a success story. The ducklings hide well enough in the night for the cat not to get one and deposit it at the foot of the stairs for me. (Nice one, black puss. Gray puss is a useless hunter and has never caught anything, which I am very grateful for.)

The next morning when I woke up, I was very reluctant to look in the shoe box as I expected the duckling to be stiff as a board with those little pleading eyes open and looking at me. You can't imagine how hard it was to lift the cover and look inside. But the cats wanted to be fed and were harassing me to get moving, which made me do it. I pulled the cover back and trying to brace myself for the expected sight of it being lifeless. Here goes. The little duckling survived the night. Yippee, and which is a very good sign that it may recover. So down my top it goes to keep warm as I had to go feed cats now.

They need warm and constant care. Each time I have rescued a duckling, they don't seem to survive if I put them somewhere overnight, like the laundry room, even though it is warm. But if they are in my bedroom, they survive. Oh well, speculation is a fun thing at times.

I love animals and I have consistently found them to be a source of peace and comfort. Yes, I think it is going to be a good day today.

CHAPTER THREE

To better understand the consequences to those left behind, I wanted to hear their stories regarding people who have committed suicide such as a parent, friend or sibling. I wanted to know what the repercussions were and what they felt both at the time and since...

I was not surprised by what I heard. The gap between understanding and not understanding why they did it is big — too big — and needs to be addressed or at least discussed with people like myself who have tried to commit suicide in earnest. As I see it, if you have the insight to something unfathomable as auctioning a plan to commit suicide, then this tiny insight may be what is needed to help with the healing process of the bereaved. Then maybe, just maybe, it will help the surviving relatives and friends to come to terms with this great sadness and perhaps understand a little of what was going on with their loved one before they died.

Well, as I was saying, these are the most common statements people made to me, but not without a little anger and sadness detected. There are surprising amounts of families who have suffered terribly and continue to do so many years later. They want to know why. There does not seem to be any closure for them. They will always have unanswered questions and pain that will not be reconciled due to the decision made by the deceased person.

People at the top end of the ladder who supposedly have everything they could possibly want in life are not immune either. When something is hurting them bad enough and they cannot face the future, they can succumb. Affluent lifestyles and power do not give protection. And for them, if they cannot talk to someone in case they look weak or incapable or whatever else, they will conjure up what seems like real reasons to them as they find they have nowhere to turn. Down the slippery slope, they can and do go to the exit door that solves all problems in their eyes, which is called suicide.

It is usually a terrible shock to loved ones, as they thought everything was fine in their life and had no reason to do such a terrible thing. With no notion as to why, people have only speculation and random guesses that may or may not come close to the reason or reasons they wanted to die. They start to think about what they should or could have done to change the situation and feel they have let them down somehow.

Alternatively, they start to speculate about all the possible clues that they could have noticed and did not. Was their behavior off in some way and they did not notice because they were too busy with their own problems? Were there any changes that they should have seen? After all, they are close to them; surely, they of all people would have known something was amiss and could have prevented them from taking their life if only they had paid a little more attention. On the other hand, they feel that maybe that fight they had last week/month with them may have been the cause.

In addition, why did they not come to them and talk about it if they were feeling bad? How could they just leave them in such a way with nothing but questions, pain and confusion as a legacy? How could they be so selfish as to just leave and not get help instead? Was there no thought or consideration about anyone else and how they would feel? It feels like a smack in the face with no apology.

The Invisible Stalker

When I talked to people who have lost someone to suicide, they tell me they are bewildered and shocked and had no understanding as to what made them do it. They loved them. They were a close family. They could think of nothing missing from their lives. They thought they had it all.

When someone close to you dies (not suicide), you go through a grieving process, and naturally for most, over time you adjust to the loss of that person. For most of us, it is painful and the grief is unbearable. But we get through it and can function once again and come to terms with it as a natural process — eventually. (Incidentally, there is an excellent book called On Death and Dying written by Dr Elizabeth Kuble-Ross . She really was a pioneer in the study of emotions we go through when we or a loved one is dying. It is worth getting from the library and having a read — you may find it a helpful guide in understanding and dealing with bereavement.

As you may imagine or sadly know, the loss of someone dear to you is very painful. However, for some families it is not quite as straightforward (if you can say such a thing!). They have to face the fact their loved one killed themselves deliberately. Well, that is an added dimension of pain to the already grieving relatives and friends. The shock and disbelief can be too much to bear at times.

For whatever reason, some families are not allowed to discuss the person who has died, which makes them feel as if their kin did not exist at all. Maybe the pain was far too great for the person who forbade them to talk about it. It is easier to bury than deal with it. Therefore, they bury it deep within themselves and expect the rest of the family to do the same.

For others, the pain doesn't really go away but can be made tolerable for these people by keeping their memory alive and not burying it. Eventually they can get great comfort from these memories and come to a place within them that makes life tolerable again thus are able to be in the now and look forward to happier times.

The knock-on effect is untold for people who have lost someone dear to them through suicide. They can become very depressed and hit a downward spiral that turns into depression, which lasts longer than it should. I personally do believe you can die of a broken heart, or perhaps that's the romantic in me! There are many stories to back this up and you probably know someone who just gave up when they lost someone through a terrible situation like suicide or murder. They spend a lifetime with that person and then they are gone, so they give up too. (Mainly the aged I am referring to here.) Just to get back up again after such a tragedy is a big step and takes time, patience and much understanding and love on our part.

I talked to one lovely woman who lost her daughter to suicide at the age of twenty-two years. She says she carries a terrible ache in her heart and there is a big void where once was a lovely, caring daughter who had everything going for her. This has scared her so much it has spilled over to her worrying about her son doing the same thing. She described him as a very quiet and sensitive boy. This fear she has just eats away at her now. She showed me photos she has on a corkboard of her two children. They look beautiful and so carefree. Who would have thought that this beautiful dark-haired girl would want to kill herself?

She says there was neither rhyme nor reason why her daughter would take her own life. She was a high achiever, outgoing, and popular. But one day, on an ordinary day like any other, her and her husband got the news.

A policeman came to the door to inform them of the tragedy. Their lovely daughter was dead. She had committed suicide. This was the only case where I did not ask what method she used. But from what the mother was saying, it was a deliberate act of taking her life.

This was a couple of years ago and since then her marriage has not survived the trauma. Their grief was so big; they couldn't talk to each other. They lost sight of each other's suffering and isolated themselves until there was nothing left for them to hold onto. They did not get counseling of any kind, but struggled on in their own grief, alone.

Another woman told me about her nephew who had committed suicide and what it did to her brother, the boy's father. He has shut him out as if he never existed. He never allows himself to think of him now. He never discusses his boy to anyone and will not have anyone talk to him about his son. His family is suffering more because there no discussions are permitted about him and they are not allowed to acknowledge his birthday or the day he died. This happened twelve years ago and he has become an angry man. He used to be a lot of fun and generally an easy going, caring kind of guy. He was very close to his son and this was completely unexpected.

What was so hard for him to take was the fact they had played footy down at the beach the day before. His son did not discuss anything with him or even hint that he had a problem of any kind. He was a happy go-lucky kid but a tad too sensitive for his own good, as his aunty puts it.

She suspected the boy was homosexual and could not tell his father as he was a "real man's man" as they say. His father was homophobic and made it known. She is only surmising this may be the real reason he took his own life. It may have seemed insurmountable to him to deal with these issues and if he had a close relationship with his father, knowing his views on homosexuality would have created a big brick wall and he probably didn't know how to get around it. Maybe but nonetheless very sad for all.

A small boy will not know his mummy, as again this child was four years old when his mother committed suicide and his grandparents are bringing him up now. But sadly, the family will not discuss her nor do they want any reminders of her around the house. She was a solo mum and very devoted to her little son. She was finding it hard on her own but did not get any help. Then one day her sister came to see her and found her. She had taken her life and left her small boy alone in the lounge.

The grandparents will not discuss their daughter to the little boy as they found it too painful, so do not mention her at all to him. His aunty said she would make sure he knows his mother when he is older and not in earshot of the rest of the family as it would be too distressing.

The most surprising story I found is because this happened many years ago and the repercussions can still be felt, closure is needed due to how it is making her feel today. This story is from a woman in her late fifties. When she realized I was writing about suicide and its effects, she opened up to me and told me her story.

She was seven and her sisters were three and five years old at the time. She remembers her mother going into the bathroom and not coming out. When someone opened the bathroom door to see how she was, they saw blood everywhere. After that, she and her sisters were shuffled into a room and made to sit on a bed with the door open so they could be kept an eye on. Otherwise they just sat there, bewildered and frightened.

People were coming and going and people wearing some sort of uniforms were taking their mother away (ambulance and police officers, I assume.) While all this chaos was going on, no one came to see if they were ok. They were ignored and not told a thing. She heard the adults talking and saying the mother had cut her wrists and throat. Again, assuming from hearing the conversations going on in the house amongst the adults. She then remembers she and her sisters being taken away and never going back home. The father was unfit to look after them himself so they went into care.

To this day, this woman is still dealing with all this. In those days, no one got counseling, let alone children! I think children were thought of as mindless, unfeeling robots that were to be quiet and did as they were told! (My of perception of course.)

She said as she gets older, she seems to get angry with her mother for doing this to them. She said it had caused so much pain and resentment and if she could talk to her mother now, she would ask her why she left three young children alone and consequently have a very hard life. Her sisters do not talk about this as she thinks they may have been a bit too young at the time to remember much, but at the age of seven years, she remembers it as if it were just yesterday.

She also remembers there was lots of trouble regarding the funeral. Because her mother was Catholic and had committed suicide, the church would not allow her to be buried in a consecrated grave. As she says, her mother has left her a legacy of heartache for the rest of her life; she is now in her late fifties and it does not get any easier. She wants to know how she could leave them and why she did it. As this woman was talking and remembering, I could see her pain and anger etched on her face. Time seems to stand still when these things happen.

I wanted to hug all these people and make the pain go away for them — me, someone who tried to do the same thing, which in turn would cause the same pain to my own children. How very insane is that? It scares and horrifies me.

There are people who experience different situations regarding the loss of someone to suicide, but the pain and confusion is what connects these people in all walks of life. I have had the privilege to hear their stories (mothers, fathers, brothers, sisters, cousins, aunties, uncles, and friends). One of the things I noted was the hesitation when they said they committed suicide.

Some were uncomfortable even saying the word suicide but wanted to get it out. In addition, one person, when asked about his son taking his life, stopped for a moment and said it leaves a bitter taste in his mouth whenever he thinks about it. He had to stop for a minute to compose himself and then carried on telling me his very sad story of his son who was twenty-two years old and had hung himself in the garage of his mother's house. They had no idea why. No clues as to what could have caused such a drastic act. He seemed fine to his family and friends. He had no girlfriend, so there were no relationship issues. Like he says, they just have to live with it and somehow try not to keep wondering why or they (he and his ex-wife) would go mad. This young man was their only son. This father says that by their son doing this, it has left them feeling broken.

One man I came across in New Zealand got chatting. When I told him I was writing a book on the depth of depression and the depth you have to go to commit suicide, he told me his story. This nice man carried his burden for many years and never told a soul about it. But it was eating away at him all that time. He said he became a workaholic, which was a good way for him to shut out the memories. He said if he stopped, he would just fall apart and never gets up again. He even contemplated suicide because of this even though he has a lovely family (two children under five years). He said he never gave them a thought at the time because he was consumed by his pain. This was the closest he ever came to this level of depression and he said quite frankly it scared him to think he could even for a minute kill himself and leave his wife and children, who he said he loved more than anything. He was raped as a kid by a "trusted adult. " He said he was about eight years old at the time. He never told anyone because his family was very God fearing and so he did not feel he could come out and say such a thing. He doubted they would have believed him and it would have only got worse for him.

Therefore, as a young boy, he felt he had to hide the fact that he was sodomised and the perpetrator was never punished for it. He said the nearest he came to being side swiped since the depression episode was when he was watching a movie called The Kite Runner. It brought a lot of very bad feelings back for him. It took him a few days to get back to "normal." (I bought the movie so I could see what he was talking about. There is a scene where a young boy is raped by this big kid. I must admit I felt very uncomfortable about it. It is not explicit, thank goodness, but you get the idea. Knowing it goes on and some victim have been scarred for life.) It was an interesting movie all the same. (Based on a true story.)

A young boy was being bullied at school. The mother did all she could to stop it. Due to the system, or inadequate solutions, it did not stop. He got very down. His mother was a solo mum; his father had died when he was young. She decided after perseverance to take him to a different school.

She let the head master know of the bullying at his previous school so he could take action if there was any more bullying. Well, there was more bullying. Again, she did what she could to get it stopped. Nothing happened and the situation did not change. The boy was getting more and more withdrawn and obviously did not want to go to school. His mother took steps she thought best to stop this from happening to her son, but sadly it did not protect him from the world of hard knocks. And it was tough on him. He got more and more depressed and withdrawn. He was going down that terrible road to what I call sub depression where there is nowhere else to go but to check out.

The young boy committed suicide. He was about fourteen years old. He left a note for his mum, saying he could not take it anymore. This terrible thing should not have happened, but it did. It gave the press something to chew over, so was publicized and for a short time there was focus on what to do about bullying in schools. Being cynical, I doubt if anything much has changed in schools since.

Therefore, that mother lost her son due to his unbearable anguish of having to go to school and being victimized by victims themselves (maybe they learned to bully from a home environment — who knows).

Here's a success story from a lovely young man in Western Australia — Aaron.

I met this young man and we talked briefly while I was traveling and doing research for this book. I met him in a beautiful part of Australia with the most amazing beaches; severance on the west coast. He was telling me about how he used to be into the drug scene with his mates. He said he started to get paranoid that people were watching him. These people looked real to him. He could not discern that they were part of his paranoia. Not only did they watch him, but they talked about all his past indiscretions and knew his guilt over everything he had done in his past!

He would look out of the window to see if he was being followed to his house. The paranoia got worse as the drugs got more frequent due to needing that "make me feel good" fix again. He started to use drugs more frequently to keep the paranoia away, which just increased cause it to increase. It was like a window of feeling OK again for a while but then the paranoia started to get worse.

He could see these people; even though they were just his delusions, they looked real to him. His thoughts turned to suicide then. He was going very quickly to a very bad place. Some of his friends had committed suicide and were into the drugs with him as well. He had the foresight to realize he was in real trouble and went to his father for help. And with the effort he put in with his father's support, he is now off the drugs and does not have the terrible paranoia and delusions. He realized it was a very close call for him. He now has a lovely son and a very good life.

Sadly, when he sees his friends, apart from declining the offer of a drug, he can see some of them doing just what he did when he was on drugs, such as getting paranoid about being followed by the police. He really feels for his friends but you have to want to stop — no one can make it happen for you. Otherwise it will not work.

He has come out of this a stronger, happier person and feels he has had a lucky escape. It was lovely to meet him and hear a success story showing him pushing through that grip of addiction, to recognize how close he had come to his demise. He got help and came through.

CHAPTER FOUR

I have heard many sad stories since researching this subject. But this was a drop-in-the-ocean sample. The question they ask seems to be the same with them all: WHY DID THEY DO IT? That alone is the most important question. But there were some nurses I spoke with and they said it would be good to know what is going on in the heads of these people who try to kill themselves. They do their job in caring for them physically but they would like to understand from a psychological point of view when they see them laying there in the hospital bed, all bandaged up from inflicted wounds and looking so lost.

As they cannot come back to tell you why they did it, you are left to wonder. I could only give them a very brief view of how I felt when I took an overdose and how I felt about it. It somehow gave them a little comfort; if such a thing can be said, knowing it was an act of a mental aberration. I told them my story the best I could. In a way, it is not their child, father, mother, etc., who was responsible for committing suicide. It had more to do with overwhelming circumstances that pushed them, and they were too far down to fight it.

I hear these people. I see the pain in their eyes as they look into the distance to hide it. I see my sons in their eyes. I see their pain too.

I listen to these people from different backgrounds and see the same sense of loss.

One young man who was mentally challenged could barely communicate, but did well enough for me to understand his loss when his best friend hung himself.

When he tells me why his friend did it, I hear the words of good therapists talking. This young man could not grasp the concept of why he died and it was explained to him in a way he could understand and accept. So he tells me in almost parrot fashion what happened for his friend to do this, and thus leave him alone. He said it happened a year ago and the doctors are helping him now. He has been put on a medication that seems to be effective. He said he liked it; it made him feel better (this is not the case for everyone, of course, but it helped this young man). He was very happy to talk about it with me and I could see he has managed to work through the grief process. But he did say he still cries sometimes. I just had to give this lovely boy a hug. Then he told me where the best fish-and-chip shop was. And he was right — the fish was wonderful.

The first time I tried to kill myself, I was beside myself with despair. I felt I had nowhere to turn. I thought my brain would explode with anguish. I remembered that long ago I had a very bad reaction to MSG (a food enhancer) and went into anaphylactic shock. The hospital did their thing and stopped the process of suffocation, which is what effectively happens with anaphylactic shock. The airways close up due to swelling and so you can't breathe. I was at the stage of this attack of anaphylaxis that I could hardly breathe and the doctor was going to do a tracheotomy if the medication did not work in time, but luckily at the time it did work and so I was spared such an experience. There were the days when I had no idea what depression was; I was not interested in knowing what it was and could not care less about such matters. (Young and green as they say, lovely!)

So, many years later, I came to the end of my endurance. I could not take anymore. I had been whittled down to a sniveling mess by this stage in my life. I thought about death and the overwhelming need for peace in my soul, let alone my life. I thought of my sons but thought they were old enough to cope. At that time I was still with my husband I so knew they had him anyway. (This was practical thinking, not a moment of emotional thinking regarding this sort of thing and the consequences.) Maybe it would have been too tough to contemplate what I would be doing to them, so I blocked it out.

I had to do something. I could no longer think of others anyway; there was nothing left inside of me that would contribute to help them with their lives now. My boys have grown up strong and confident. I just hoped their father would be able to continue to nurture and support the children as needed. I had nothing left inside of me.

I thought again about MSG, this way would look like an accident, I thought. So there would be no extra burden to carry, knowing their mother killed herself. It drags up too many incorrect reasons. So a nice clean death due to allergy reaction and asphyxiation would be respectable.

I went to the Asian shop looking for MSG and eventually found some in the supermarket. It is a white power and you don't need much to do the job if you are already allergic to it (or anything, for that matter). So I came home and put the whole tin in a can of coke and drank it.

Then I thought I needed to get my heart rate up sufficiently to make it work faster. I did a jog up the hill behind my house, which is part of my land, so if I did go into shock, I would not be found until I was well and truly cold and not revivable. So I jogged up the hill, thinking the jogging was going to kill me never mind the MSG. I felt my heart pumping faster and I was sweating from the effort of this physical workout that I had not done in many a year! The body did protest with my lungs burning and throat sore, but I pushed myself. Then I could not move one more step. I fell down in the grass and lay there, breathing hard and looking at the sky, which was looking like it might rain as there was a thick layer of cloud.

As I lay there waiting for the tingling to start in my face, this is where it started before, along with crazy itching and coughing. (Well, you cough the breath out as this is the only way the body can expel the air from the lungs as it squeezes shut — a normal reaction that kicks in for survival.)

I lay there for two hours. I already realized it was not going to work. It should have started to work more or less immediately after taking the stuff. I could not believe it. I stood up and screamed and cursed the sky (not sure what that could have achieved). I exercised a few swear words too, which I don't usually do. It made no difference. All my screaming and shouting at the gods and cosmos did not change a thing. I was still here. But the ducks got a good show. I just crumpled up in the grass and cried.

After a while when I was all spent, I went back to the house and got in the bath for a few hours (that's the only place I can get privacy and time out from my husband who I am sure is ADHD). When I turned into a wrinkly prune and had goose bumps on goose bumps, I slowly got out of the bath, feeling emotionally washed out and exhausted. With what energy I had left I dried myself and dressed. I went downstairs where my husband and sons were in the TV room I went into the room and sat down and pretended to watch TV and to carry on with my life as if nothing had happened. I had to get through another day.

The second time I tried to commit suicide was so ironic. I took an overdose this time, knowing the amount of pills I took would sink a battleship and I knew these were bad pills. I knew these would work. I went to bed after taking them, thinking this time; this time it is going to work. I was in a terrible place, so much so I wanted to kill myself and at last I can. That is the bottom line. I was on my own now. The house was empty. I did not expect visitors for a while so had at least a few days clearance to be too long gone for intervention.

I lay in bed with a big sigh of relief and waited for sleep or death, whichever came first, and then that would be it, the end of me. I must have fallen asleep quite quickly. There will be no more me. No more emotional punch bag. The punch bag will be out of commission forever. I was escaping life's wrath.

But I woke up the next morning. I was confused, first of all. I knew something was to have happened, and then it dawned on me: I should have been dead. I could not believe it. What the hell was going on with my body? Why is it still living? I took sixty something pills that are known to kill in small doses. It should have worked. There is no doubt. I cried.

I thought then that there must be a God and he/she is playing with me. Waiting to see what happens when I can't escape life. I thought I was being punished extra cruelly. So much for being mortal. I felt my body was going to go on forever which scared me to death, unintended pun there! I was so down about still being me I phoned a friend who has suffered depression and has been there for me through this tough stuff. He is a very sensitive person and has such understanding and empathy. I told him what I did and that it had not worked. He was horrified, of course, but said these particular pills do not work this way. They take days to work. They slowly destroy your liver and kidneys and it is a slow and painful death. I was so relieved to hear this. I thought I was immune to death itself!

So there really is going to be an end to my depression after all. I just had to be patient. Of course, my friend was now worried about me and begged me to go to the hospital as they can reverse this drug if done in time. The window of opportunity is small for this procedure. Of course, I said no way and that he has to keep my confidence as I have for him. I was emotionally blackmailing him, I suppose. But I desperately needed him to understand I could not go on anymore. I told him that when he confided in me about stuff, I kept his confidence. This was payback time. I needed him to understand my pain as only he could, as he had been where I am now. Over a few hours of talking, I think he realized I had had enough and cannot go on anymore. I was serious. I also told him he was being a wonderful friend and this is what I wanted. I wanted him to understand and remember the terrible pain depression can bring and I have had far too much of it for a few lifetimes. I wanted to quit. I was happy to quit. Finito. Give in. Crawl away. Whatever way you want to describe what I am doing is OK with me. I don't care. I have had it. He had to understand this and respect my wishes to die. I eventually put the phone down after what I thought was a good convincing argument as to why he had to hold my confidence. I immediately felt relief. I was leaving this hell hole for good. (I never at any time thought it would adversely affect my sons and they would be OK. Plus I had a fat insurance policy they would benefit from.) Oh I was so practical. I was incapable of thinking they may suffer from my death. Denial maybe. I don't know. I just know financially they will be OK. And they are grown up. Interestingly enough, I never had parents when I was grown up so I don't know the advantages they bring to your life. So I could not comprehend something I never had, for my boys.

So after convincing Aaron that I am doing what I want and it is ok for me, we ended our call. I felt a little guilty afterwards because Aaron is a lovely friend and I did not want to put this on his head. I think I did a good job though, and maybe he understood a little. So I go and have a bath (again) it is my security blanket I think. I work out then who I could get to come to the house to cart me away before my son comes home and finds me. I decided to write a note to the ambulance station and by the time it gets there, it should be ok. Yes, good idea. I then get into the bath.

My son turns up at my house very worried a half hour after I got off the phone with my friend. My friend had phoned my son but did not tell him I took an overdose but said I needed some extra medication at the emergency department and it was urgent. My son could not understand why my friend was crying, so he got very worried about me and came to my house to see me.

I was not expecting this and I had to think quickly as I did not want my son to know what I had done and also not to let anything interrupt the process of the drugs destroying my organs. So I said yes, I had to get a B12 shot sometimes at the doctor's as my medication was not being as effective as it should. But no biggie, I would attend to it sometime in the week. But from the look on his face and my track record with depression, I don't think he believed me, but was not sure what was really going on.

He said I might as well go get the B12 shot rather than put it off until later in the week. Then it will make me feel much better. I could see he was not going to budge until I did this, so said I agreed to go to the hospital and do this but would rather take my own car (otherwise my son would escort me to the hospital to make sure I did it). He said that was OK and he would follow in his car back to town. Great, I thought, once he turns off at his road, I will just turn my car around and come back home without going to the hospital.

So my son followed behind my car all the way to the hospital when I thought he would turn off for home. I parked at the hospital, but so did my son. I got out of my car and went to where he was parked and said there was no point in him coming in with me, as it is only a routine injection and that is no big deal for me. He said OK, he would not come in then. Great, I thought, now I can go, just as soon as he drives away. But no, he stood there and was not budging until I went in the doors, which are all glass. He could see then if I went into the reception area. When I got to the reception desk, which I did not want to get to, as I had no intention of letting them know I took an overdose, I asked the nurse if my son who was wearing a blue jacket was still outside the doors. He said yes. So I turned around and waved, my son waved back and carried on leaning on his car with his arms folded. He was not going anywhere. He did not trust me. Surprise surprise.

So obviously I could not say to the nurse I was there for a B12 shot as they don't do this sort of thing when someone just turns up at the accident and emergency department, where I was. So I had to come clean. I said I took some pills and before I could say any more, the nurse said, oh, it is you. Yes, we know all about it. And so I was whisked away into the chasm of the healing centre for treatment to reverse the effects. My friend who lives in another part of the country phoned them for information about the timeframe I had before it was irreversible. So that was how they already knew about me.

Because I took the drugs longer than twenty-four hours prior, they would not be in the stomach so could not be pumped out thus they have to give me something to counteract the effects. Then they made me get onto the bed (after putting their lovely gowns on, of course; the ones that show off your bottom if you try to make a break for it).

I was wired up, pricked, pumped, questioned (none to do with my state of mind, of course; they were dealing with the body only). It took about an hour for them to do blood work, get results to see the type of drugs I used and how much, I suppose, and then calculate how much of this solution to hook me up to. After all was done, they hooked me up to the intravenous solution to reverse the effects and stop my organs from being destroyed. It is hell not getting away from the mental torture as the nurses and doctors automatically keep you alive.

But irony of irony, I was allergic to the solution. When the young nurse was pushing my bed to a cubicle while the solution was flowing into my veins, I could feel the familiar sensation that told me I was starting to react to the solution they were using. When this happens, my face goes red and swells up quite a bit and then I start to cough — the anaphylaxis cough. So there were obvious external signs that could tell the world I was going into shock. So I kept my head down as if I was crying with my hands covering my face. But the cough is so hard to suppress even though I tried to cough quietly (try stopping a coughing fit — it is impossible. Same for the cough I was experiencing where my body was trying to expel air from my lungs that was being closed off).

But unfortunately the nurse looked up from where she was plugging in monitors to the wall in the cubicle and saw for herself my blotchy, swollen face (I couldn't see by this stage as my eyes where squashed shut by the skin around my eyes).

All I could deduce was she had realized what was happening and called stat and I was being rushed to the resuscitation room. They had the injections ready and waiting. So they stopped the anaphylactic shock by giving the magic potion that does that job well.

As all this busyness was going on around me, I still couldn't see, but I was thinking of the irony of this situation when not so long ago I tried to induce anaphylaxis and it did not work — hmmm!

But then I realized, hey, I am allergic to this reversal solution, so does that mean they cannot reverse the drugs I took? Hmmmm. No, they were not giving up on me, even if I had. They diluted the solution with saline and gave it to me over sixteen hours, which is very slow. This worked. I did not go into shock.

Then my son was talking to me. I still couldn't see, as it takes awhile for swelling to go down. He was amazed by my face. I told him I got a reaction from the B12 shot. I did not want him to know what I had done. Why stress out my boy when I don't have to, right?

Of course, they had no intentions of letting me go home

and now my son was there so I had to do more thinking and conniving and lying. I was not going to let anyone tell my boy the truth.

The staffs at the hospital (Dunedin Public) really do a good job and they are very ethical as far as patient confidentiality goes. I told them at the earliest opportunity to make sure no nurse, doctor, cleaner or anyone talked to my son about my situation. Even out of desperation, I quoted a few rights of the patients but they know their job and were very good. They made him leave the room if they had to ask any pertinent questions about my state of mind and overdose.

I told my son my meds were not very good and I may be having them changed, so I might have to stay in the hospital while I came off one type and onto another. I knew I had to stay in. You don't stay in the hospital just because you have had a reaction to a B12 shot, which is what my son thinks. So more thinking, more side stepping the issue with my son, and I came up with this brilliant plausible reason why I would be going to the emergency psychiatric ward. (Yes, I think you go stupid when you're trying to pull the wool over peoples eyes!)

You know something, even though I thought I had it all covered where my son was concerned (thank goodness my other son was overseas working at the time) but my dear boy knew what I did. He did not let on. He allowed me to think I was saving his feelings. He was so strong for me and allowed my delusions until I was ready to tell him myself, which I did eventually, but he realized from the beginning and put the pieces together himself and came up with the obvious.

CHAPTER FIVE

I want to highlight the force of our survival skills. But, for some of us, well, we seem to have something working against this instinct. (Maybe a bit of rust in the works, clogging things up!) In a way, we are stuck in our heads with our nightmares being the jailer. I am stating the obvious here, but it needs to be stated. People don't commit suicide for no reason. So, of course they don't do it for selfish reasons; that is "normal thinking" as opposed to abnormal thinking and that happens in the suicidal zone of thoughts.

Personally, I think the hormones have a lot to answer for! They can send you on a roller coaster ride of your life (drugs, for instance). Horror films, hormonal imbalance can set you up with your own horror show. You become the actor and the viewer because you can scare yourself to death!

The survival instincts are amazing and it usually works without you thinking about it, like swerving on some ice on the road. Your reaction is quicker than you can think about it. You can probably remember occasions where you have acted so fast to avert something bad, like the skidding on the road. It is strong; it is fast; it is like calling up a super power thinking to act quickly when needed. When you have eaten something off, the body rebels and throw it out of the body and for good measure, all the white blood cells come calling to make sure there is nothing left in the body that could hurt you. We have an array of support systems in us to keep us alive and safe. And funny enough, your average Joe blows have no idea how it all works, but it is our body…it is like the mind. We think we know how our own minds work, but most of us don't until something pushes us to find out how much more there is to learn about it and the adverse effects it can have on us.

When we sense danger, our bodies automatically go into alert mode by releasing more adrenaline into the bloodstream in an effort to ensure a more acute awareness of the situation facing us so we can react quickly to avert the danger. For example, walking across the road and in that second, see a car coming. In that second, our internal system has taken in the car, distance to you, assessed the safety distance from the car, realized we need to move fast, and hay presto; we sprint to the safety of the pavement. We do so automatically, unaware of our brain working to keep us safe. So we aren't run over by the car. You automatically protect yourself from dangers that present themselves. When you are well and healthy, you do not think of killing yourself. You are thinking of the next pay check so you can go out with your mates, or the next rugby game to watch the all blacks and expect them to win by a big margin! Or just doing what you do that carries you through your day. You are doing what you are supposed to do. Living, doing, and getting the most out of life. No matter how tough the environment, you want to survive — to live.

The instinct for survival is ultimately the strongest we have. This includes all living things on this planet. You try standing on an ant; it will try to run to save itself. The wild animals instinctively know to fear man, as we represent death to them. (We really are the Grim Reapers on this planet!)

Let me ask you these questions. I want to have you think about this and maybe a door will open for you to look further into the whys of such tragedies. They say knowledge is power, but in this case knowledge is a balm to help you move forward. Please think about the questions, as they are not insignificant in such matters as this. It is the path many have taken for reasons only known to them.

Would you want to take an overdose?
 Would you want to slit your wrists?
Would you want to hang yourself?

Then maybe you would want to suffocate in toxic fumes until you're dead?
What about putting a gun to your head and pulling the trigger?

Of course, the answer should be a resounding no.

It is an awful thing to contemplate, isn't it, but people not only contemplate it, they follow through.

The next question is do you think children get so depressed that they kill themselves? (I am talking from around the age of eleven years old.)

Shockingly, the answer is yes.

I have heard even younger than eleven, but have not found out for myself about younger. How can a child have gotten to the depth of hell at such a tender age? They haven't any experience with the harshness that life can dish out yet, or have they? That applies to teenagers too.

Why are they getting younger and younger? Are they being selfish too? (Doesn't the word selfish that is banded about seem out of place here?) So why do people say it often when someone takes their own life?

The Invisible Stalker

What can possibly drive them to this extreme action?
Why didn't they talk about it?
Why didn't they think of their families and how they would feel?
Why would they do this if they were happy and outgoing?
Why kill yourself and leave your child all alone in the same house? (This does happen.)

Talking is the easiest thing to do when there are no real problems in your life! Talking is the hardest thing to do it seems when there are big problems in your life!
Why is that?
If we could talk freely without any risk of condemnation or critics or misunderstanding or conditioning through upbringing, etc., then it would be easy, right?

It seems that the more serious our problems are, and we need some kind of help to deal with it, we tend to stay quiet — why is that?

Maybe we are hoping it will dissolve in the night, like magic. Wouldn't that be great?

No such luck. We have to face things, big and small, and generally, we can. We all have battle scars to prove it too. But just sometimes, that doesn't happen.

Well let me ask the next question, what emotionally stable person that you know of has taken their life? (I emphasize emotionally stable and this does not include euthanasia for terminal illness.)

Emotionally stable people do not go out and just jump off bridges because they are having an off day.

It is a buildup over time (short or long period). Selfish

people? Attention seekers? Vengeful people? They may be selfish so-and-so's but, if they are emotionally stable, selfish people don't top themselves. They would be too worried in case they missed out on something to their advantage. (Excuse the flippancy.)

These are the comments I hear often. I did try to kill myself and I know I am none of those things. (Well, we all have elements but not to this degree.)

So, no is the answer. They would not kill themselves if they were healthy individuals! However, very sick people would, and do so, with mental and physical illnesses.

You have to be privy to the depth of depressive hell where suicidal thoughts are born. Only people with problems, real or imagined, eventually overwhelm them, go down that path.

Now you can slit your wrists if you are in that depressive hellhole because it seems to be the best and most logical solution at the time. (You really believe this when you're down there. The logic is all upside down.)

This incidentally reminds me of when I was in the emergency psychiatric ward as a patient. (No, it is not a scary place, honest.) I talked to this young girl who was there for her own mental traumas. She looked no more than about eighteen years old.

She was a tiny, pretty girl with big blue eyes that looked so sad. She should have been anywhere else but there. There were more young people there than older ones. (Like the mall — sorry girls, I don't really know what eighteen-year-olds do nowadays, but I used to go ice skating a lot or dancing. Those were the good times

The Invisible Stalker

before I knew what the word mental health was all about.) She had the most awful scars up both her arms. They weren't surface scars, like when you scratch yourself badly and it heals into a little silver line to show where the scratch was. These scars were a livid pinky-purple color and raised like a mountain range down her arms from up near her elbows. There were quite a few of these jagged lines that were like a gauge indicating pain tolerance levels. I asked how she got them, assuming she would say something like a car accident or bike accident, I didn't expect what she did say.

She was very matter of fact about it and was quite happy to explain why she did such a thing. She said that the mental pain could get so bad she would want to get away from it but couldn't and so she would get a cup or saucer, smash it on the floor, then get a jagged piece and slowly cut her arms because when she was down in the "bad place," as she puts it, the cutting of her arms dulled the "mental" pain for a while and she could cope better with physical pain than that mental "stuff. "

I assumed it released endorphins (a happy hormone) when she did this, which helped her cope. It is a drastic thing to do, but at least she was alive and had the chance to work on her illness with medical help.

I must say I was shocked as she was so young to do such brutal things to her body. In addition, she seemed too young and unworldly to have built up a portfolio of bad experiences to get her into this state of depression. Then, as we are slowly finding out, there are too many children out there that find out quickly about the brutality of men/women and these children are defenseless to stop it happening to them and so have to take whatever is thrown at them in silence. By the time they grow older and wiser, the damage is done. (Beatings, rape, sodomy, I can think of as starters.) What really goes on out there on this perfect-looking planet of ours? Now I have a better understanding of why she did it. I had to get to that bad place myself to know.

Ironically, about a year or so later, I had a very bad time and was so agitated; I cut all my hair off! I had longish hair then. The support team was lovely as usual and said that was definitely preferable to the other option I could have taken.

CHAPTER SIX

It is about time this subject is really out in the open instead of behind closed doors or Chinese whispers. There is always a sense of shame and shock. Yes, this stupid stigma needs to be vanquished to the pits of hell where it belongs. And yes, I have been told clearly by so-called "authoritarian" people (not referring to medical professionals, of course) that it is a very selfish act and they would be punished in the afterlife. (I did refrain from shoving a candle up his haughty orifice!)

There were one or two bigots I came across when researching this. I am not going to do battle with them; they are too indoctrinated and would not hear my words anyway.

The majority of decent, ordinary people like you are open to a better understanding of this mental illness. Then you will truly know it is an illness, and one that can be cured or managed just like other mental illnesses are cured or managed if caught in time. But sadly, some people fall through the gaps.

Life's road is at the best of times a tough road to travel, with higher expectations and a faster pace of life. So for us who just find it too tough at times to keep up with the pressures, we fall and sometimes fall so far down that we can't get up again.

Most of us have at one time or another thought of jumping off a bridge when things got tough, but bounced back quick enough to think they were crazy to even think such a thing!

We can, at times, be a very tough people to please and

the expectation seems to get tougher and harder to achieve when you are on the downside of life for whatever reason. We sometimes are quick to show condescension rather than understanding; look the other way rather than give a helping hand. If we look, we see someone sinking and continue on our way. We have are own problems, right? (Forgive me if it seems I am preaching; it is not intended, but just pointing out some common habits of us mere mortals.) So sometimes when we need the understanding and patience the most, we find ourselves alone either by choice or the world is too busy to stop and listen to you and your miserable whining; a contributing factor that makes life even tougher for some of us. So we find an outlet in many ways like alcohol, drugs, gambling, aggression, self-mutilation, and then when there is nothing left, your emotions, your screwed-up logic takes you on that one-way journey to suicide.

You really believe there is nowhere to turn and you feel ashamed to have to ask for help. You are at the end of the road.

There seems to be a morbid curiosity with suicide from the spectator's view. When, say, a celebrity is getting hounded to crazy Dom, the tabloids hint that they may commit suicide and wait with heightened expectation for them to top themselves.(I am thinking of that young girl, Britney Spears, as an example). The tabloids were ruthless with her. I think the majority of decent people were very concerned for her (who read these magazines, like me) but felt that no one was helping her when she needed it the most. But where was the help? What was the camera crew thinking when they were taking photos of this young girl on the sidewalk breaking down in tears. Dollars, right? She had lost her babies in a custody battle to her husband. She was put under a microscope and her problems splashed on front covers of magazines around the world. Did anyone protect her from the photographers? How would they like it if their child was in that situation and being banded around the world for nosey people like me to read over a cup of tea?

But in the end they did not get their big story of her going over the edge, so they could rehash her life story and find people to blame for it and sell to the highest bidder. No, this young girl made it. She made it on her own. She was able to pull herself out of that dark place and recover to her full, beautiful, talented self. And now the tabloids are not quite so interested in her. Hmm!

The assumption that the person looks miserable and moans about how rotten his or her life is and wants to jump off a bridge is no indicator of how he or she really feels. It is easy to recognise someone who suffers from bad depression but sometimes it is not that easy. There are definite things to look out for.

We can start to understand this illness and maybe get some help for those who really need it. It is only when you lose someone to suicide that you realise its brutality. Prevention is the cure. By being more tuned into the signs and symptoms, there can be help for one of your kin.

There may be someone that you suspect has a problem?

CHAPTER SEVEN

NEGATIVE THOUGHTS TAKE YOU TO A BAD PLACE
AND SOMETIMES DO NOT LET YOU GO.

Over time, the problem, which is causing this distress,
could be anything at all. If it is consuming the mind 24/7
and is negative, it can be disruptive to you and your
family. Then these negative thoughts take you to a
worse place, in a dungeon, alone with no door handles
on the inside. This place is your worst fears and
paranoia and so the worse you feel, the less
communicative, the bigger the trap. Because I think it is
a trap. It lulls you into thinking all the pain and anguish
and everything else that has got on top of you over the
years will vanish. That becomes the focus. There is no
peripheral vision. You just focus on this release. Nothing
else exists. It is as if the mind shuts anything else out.
(Well I should say the cancer of the mind shuts
everything else out.) That's why I think if you get a note
they were cognitive enough to try to explain why they
had to go, but that is not an easy thing to do. I know I
am being very presumptuous, but after talking to people
who have survived regarding their thoughts just before
the deadly deed; their thoughts seemed to be identical
to mine. You are unable to voice your worries. It is silent
in the darkness and you don't ask or indicate that you
need help. You become almost reclusive. There is a
feeling of inertia. I have been there once too often
myself. It is not a welcoming place to be. Although it is a
self-imposed exile by the troubled mind, it is also
powerful enough for you not to recognize the state you
are in. You just had to escape the mental torture and it
was the only solution. Nothing else exists but that.

When the seemingly only conclusion is to commit

suicide, you feel a great sense of relief. It is as if you came up with the correct equation to a complicated puzzle and found the right answer to release you from the torture chamber. It is a death trap. You are so convinced that you are doing the right thing that you are ok about it. This is a major aberration. You really do not recognize the dangerous road you are on.

I am not talking about minor depression where you can recover independently of any additional support. But this level is like a sublevel, if you like. It is a one-way door to hell. The problem, which could seem minor to one person, becomes this huge insurmountable problem to another. This is where you get your ticket to hell. This is the level where suicides take place. Unless you have been there, you cannot know its grip on your mind, body and soul. It consumes you until you barely know who you are anymore or what your purpose is in life. I guess I am understating this fact, but this is the best I can do to demonstrate the fixation suicidal people have on the belief of a utopia suicide may bring. Or a cessation of pain. I can attest to the enormousness of the emotional pain; I would only wish it on Hitler if he were still alive. It may take years to get to this stage, or just a very short time. I was the former. The thing is we seem to be incapable of asking for help. It is like a weakness to do so. Or an embarrassment, or too big a quest for help. So dumb!

Reference from A.D.A.M.
A.D.A.M., Inc. is accredited by URAC, also known as the American Accreditation HealthCare Commission (www.urac.org). URAC's accreditation program is an independent audit to verify that A.D.A.M. follows rigorous standards of quality and accountability. A.D.A.M. is among the first to achieve this important distinction for online health information and services.

Learn more about A.D.A.M.'s editorial policy, editorial process and privacy policy. A.D.A.M. is also a founding member of Hi-Ethics and subscribes to the principles of the Health on the Net Foundation (www.hon.ch).

Causes

Suicidal behaviors can accompany many emotional disturbances, including depression, bipolar disorder, and schizophrenia. More than 90 percent of all suicides are related to a mood disorder or other psychiatric illness.

Suicidal behaviors often occur in response to a situation that the person views as overwhelming, such as social isolation, death of a loved one, emotional trauma, serious physical illness, aging, unemployment or financial problems, guilty feelings, or dependence on alcohol or other drug.

In the U.S., suicide accounts for about 1 percent of all deaths each year. The elderly have the highest rate of suicide, but there has been a steady increase among adolescents. Suicide is now the third leading cause of death for fifteen- to nineteen-year-olds, after accidents and homicide.

Suicide attempts that do not result in death far outnumber completed suicides. Many unsuccessful suicide attempts are carried out in a manner that makes rescue possible. These attempts often represent a desperate cry for help.

The method of suicide can be relatively nonviolent (such as poisoning or overdose) or violent (such as shooting oneself). Males are more likely to choose violent methods, which probably accounts for the fact that suicide attempts by males are more likely to be completed. Many suicides involve a firearm. This is especially true in elderly men, in which 80 percent of suicides are performed with a gun.

Relatives of people who seriously attempt or complete suicide often blame themselves or become extremely angry, seeing the attempt or act as selfish. However, when people are suicidal, they often mistakenly believe that they are doing their friends and relatives a favor by taking themselves out of the world. These irrational beliefs often drive their behavior.

Symptoms

Early signs:
Depression
Statements or expressions of guilt feelings
Tension or anxiety
Nervousness
Impulsiveness

Critical signs:
Sudden change in behavior, especially calmness after a period of anxiety
Giving away belongings, attempts to "get one's affairs in order"
Direct or indirect threats to commit suicide
Direct attempts to commit suicide

Treatment
Emergency measures may be necessary after a person has attempted suicide. First aid, CPR, or mouth-to-mouth resuscitation may be required.

Hospitalization is often needed to treat the recent actions and to prevent future attempts. Psychiatric intervention is one of the most important aspects of treatment.

Expectations (prognosis)

Suicide attempts and threats should always be taken seriously. About one-third of people who attempt suicide will repeat the attempt within one year, and about 10 percent of those who threaten or attempt suicide eventually do kill themselves.

Mental health care should be sought immediately. Dismissing the person's behavior as attention-seeking can have devastating consequences.

Complications

Complications vary depending on the type of suicide attempt.

Calling Your Health Care Provider

A person who threatens or attempts suicide MUST be evaluated immediately by a mental health professional. NEVER IGNORE A SUICIDE THREAT OR ATTEMPT!

Prevention

Many people who attempt suicide talk about it before making the attempt.

Sometimes, simply talking to a sympathetic, non-judgmental listener is enough to prevent the person from attempting suicide. For this reason, suicide prevention centers have telephone "hotline" services. Again, do not ignore a suicide threat or attempted suicide.

As with any other type of emergency, it is best to immediately call the local emergency number. Do not leave the person alone even after phone contact with an appropriate professional has been made.

For those of you who have access to the Internet, this is

a good site for more information.
http://health.nytimes.com/health/guides/disease/suicide-and-suicidal-behavior/overview.html

CHAPTER EIGHT

Take myself, for instance. I come across as a very bubbly, happy-go-lucky individual. In a way, it is hard not to judge a book by it's cover sometimes as our lives are very busy and there is just not the time. I would be judged by my cover and understandably so as I do portray an upbeat kinda gal. Many years ago, someone said to me that if your happy, people would be nice to you, and somehow it stuck and I took this on as a front and a protection. It is not so easy to be aggressive to a "happy" person as it is to a grumpy person. My thinking and philosophy. This is partly because over the years I have become so ashamed of these feelings of inadequacy I have. I cannot bear to think that people will find out that I get depressed so I go over the top when it comes to my outward appearance. If you're happy, you're not depressed, right? I think people will judge me and make me feel even more isolated than I already felt. Having depression can have the effect of forcing you into isolation to lick your wounds and hide. I used many guises to do this.

One was to go to the cinema — this sounds odd, but it is a place where I can hide. It is dark and you are not recognized thus avoid conversation. The other was the swimming pool where I would take a book and sit there pretending to read just to make sure no one talked to me. I could not go home, as that was a very bad place for me when I was going down. The triggers are big at home. Therefore, it had to be a public place, which made me feel "safe," and I could isolate myself verbally at the same time. There is a bonus to this method, as there was mental stimulation from external sources, and you had to hold it together long enough for the feelings to subside — or bad thoughts, that is. All the people who have committed suicide become infested with the bad thoughts that start to overtake them, and this is so not good because they die. That is why I have to be in a public place before the bad thoughts take over. These worked well for me. Usually, I am drained by the time I do go home as it is quite exhausting to fight the monster.

Intervention, education, medication, changes to habits and revaluation of what is important; all these things have a part to play in getting back to recovery. And sometimes they can feel even better than they have in years.

For those who have had depression and those who are fighting depression, they know it is not an easy feat to overcome this monster without constant and exhaustive work on oneself. (Pushing water up hill is a preferable option, and would be easier at times!) However, sometimes you have to do whatever it takes to keep the mood swings at a manageable level.

Just like other illnesses, take alcoholism, for instance, they can never have another alcoholic drink because they know the power this digression can have on them and they would soon find themselves controlled by this awful demon that demands they have another drink and another... They know they cannot take this road, even for a moment so have to avoid any temptations for the rest of their lives. There is no reprieve.

I could not trust myself when I was crashing, and the family knows this. You can get quite devious when you want to escape the torment of the mind. I wanted to run away from myself, which is impossible to do (there you go and there you still are. This was someone's quote from a book but can't remember who — so apt!).

Moreover, the only escape I could think of was to sleep it away (forever), which was not the right solution due to the repercussions on my family and friends. So the only way I had at the time to help me be somewhere safe, even if only psychologically, was I drew a picture of this boat, which took me to this island, and it crumbled in the effort to get me there…(I drew a bird or two, well, not that they look like birds, but with a little imagination, and the canvas at a distance of 100 meters away, it could look like a bird to keep me focused on beauty in the world).

The drawing still came out quite somber looking but this was the best I could do with the way I felt. (No rainbows, no sunny days, no pretty flowers, as they were too far up the ladder of happiness for me to visualize.) This is how I felt as I was painting the picture; it was sheer effort to create this picture to enable me to feel free, surrounded by nature.

Sometimes this works well if I have the materials ready. I usually keep a supply of canvas and paints (from the two-dollar shop!) so it is not expensive to do. This practice helps me get through a bad time by visualizing myself in the picture, or identifying with it…

*I have put the pictures at the end of the book with a brief description of what they mean to me.

The next picture, for example, I did when I was feeling particularly agitated and needed to be alone, but it was not possible at the time. I was going through a tough time keeping the depression at bay, so the family did not let me out of their sight, understandably. (I think they call it suicide watch, sad to say.) Therefore, the next best thing was to draw a retreat for myself so that I could be alone and be safe at the same time.

The Invisible Stalker

When I finished it, it had done two things for me: Firstly, it kept me occupied while I fought with negative feelings about myself. In addition, as people know who have to fight depression, it is quite exhausting both emotionally and physically. Secondly, the act of painting and being focused was soothing and calmed me until I got through this and started to feel the anxiety lifting. I don't want to talk to anyone when I am feeling bad, so when the family wants to know how I am feeling I almost always verbalize with one or two syllables as I find it hard to string sentences together when I am depressed. Therefore, I am left to paint or draw until I can lift my mood to a manageable level.

That was how I felt when things were becoming too much in the end. I was feeling a sense of inadequacy. I should have been able to cope, so I thought. I was ashamed to contemplate telling anyone I could not cope anymore. Imagine what they would think. I felt useless. I worried it was a massive dose of self-pity. I did not want people feeling sorry or pitying me. That would just make things worse. This sense of inadequacy I think was the worst for me. Now, as you can see, I thought people would think all these negative things about me and rather than face that I tried to deal with my problems alone and without telling anyone. This is the problem in general. We try to cope on our own. I did and it did not work; the feelings only got worse. After all, you see people around you with worse problems and they cope. We usually bear the burden alone. Nevertheless, sometimes, someone out there just hits the wall, as I did. It does happen, more than it should. This does not include people with chemical imbalance; they are in their own category.

We seem to have these preconceived ideas that if you're not strong or able minded, you're worthless and thus condemned by society. Of course, this is not the case. Maybe it is from way back in the cave-dweller days when they beat you over the head with a thigh bone for your meat because they can! Who knows but we do find it hard to bear our souls and ask for help. Especially, I think men have a much harder time opening up. I personally think they have a harder time opening up than women do. So in a way, our problems are not just the problem itself, but also communication, the lack of. This is the root cause in a way; if the problem is out in the open and not stuck in your head growing into a monster problem, it can become less controlling in a much healthier way. Maybe with a little help, and help is indeed a good thing.

As some of you realize, when we have a problem, it always seems smaller when we talk about it than when it is just in our heads. Now that is not downplaying the seriousness of something, but it is just easier to deal with when it is out there (i.e. I am not talking about putting it in the newspapers or anything; I was thinking more of a doctor, which is the best place to start as they refer you to the right people, like a good councilor or someone you trust.)

There are more caring people out there than I ever thought possible before I had my eyes opened.

As far as suicide notes, the people who did get them were the "fortunate" ones showing explanations, but quite a few do not write a note. Now I can certainly understand why they don't write a note. When you reach that level of depression, notes are not on the agenda; hell, nothing but escape is on the agenda. Getting away from the pain is the most important thing to do, whatever it takes. I didn't think of a note when I took a massive overdose (three times). I mentally thought of my boys, of course, but in a "practical way" very unemotional and robotic is a good way to describe it. I thought about things like do I have enough life insurance and do they know who the lawyer is. Those sort of practicalities, as you would if you were going on a long holiday. That was the essence of this organizing of the affairs.

So maybe because I did not leave a note, it did not compute in my brain to do so. Maybe it was a denial of what I was doing. I don't know and am only guessing. I know how important it is for the bereaved to have had a note of some kind to explain why. From memory and my notes I made during the depressive episodes, I was finding life very difficult and could not see a future. There seemed to be no way out of this and I was convinced I would always be struggling to keep above the depression. I felt as if I was totally against the wall, as they say.

Then the depression got worse to the level of blinding me of any other options open to me. Apathy, fear, anxiety and sense of failure have been my constant companion to a greater or lesser degree.

For example, I would get very anxious when I smelled a certain perfume. The sense of smell is powerful. It can trigger you to recall all sorts of things from the past that is associated with that particular smell. This perfume brought back very bad memories for me, which I had not dealt with (post-traumatic stress disorder). The anxiety was present day, but the root cause was much earlier in my life. Moreover, until I deal with it, it will continue to haunt me.

CHAPTER NINE

I want to give you an idea of what went on in my head, and the powerful emotions I experienced at the time, which accumulated in me taking a massive overdose that should have killed me.

This troubled mind of mine was taking me down that road to committing suicide and I could not recognize the danger I was in at first, and then it was too late. It is a mental illness that should have been treated by a health professional, as it was too complex for me to even understand, never mind deal with alone (unrealized the time).

I have been in decline emotionally over the years and my defenses are getting thinner by the day. Therefore, when I have a bad day, there is not much reserve left to protect me from the depression I kept falling into. The only trouble was that the depression was getting deeper and deeper until it was nearly impossible to get out of. I knew I had to stay alive for my children all these years. It was my only focus. I had to be there for them until they were adults. So I won the fight each time when I thought of my children being motherless and not having me there as they grew up. I hung on with super determination to not let the depression overwhelm me because frankly I would have gladly died if I did not have the boys to care for.

But then my lovely boys had grown into wonderful young men. My reserves had gotten weaker as they grew confident and capable. I knew they were grown and could manage without me. Therefore, I knew I was vulnerable. However, I still did not recognize the fact I needed help. I did not realize just how low my reserves were.

It seemed like another ordinary day; it may have been a weekend. My oldest son was at his house. My youngest son was overseas. I fed the cats and then checked on the ducks outside. All seemed well, apart from my demons sitting on my shoulder all the time, which retrospectively I should have been on my guard about. It was not unusual for me to be below par as this is in a way normal for me. But this day I had my self-worth battered again and I think this was the last straw.

I walked into a brick wall, metaphorically speaking. I felt sick inside and my heart was still pounding as I tried to control the escalation downward. It is like a panic attack; I needed to get off this planet. I just could not cope one more day here. I had no self-esteem, which was eroded over the years, and no self-preservation kicking in to stop this self-attack.

Slowly my traumatized mind went into overdrive and this is where the poles reverse. What you think is self-protection and is right is actually self-destruction and so wrong. This is how I feel when I am having a very bad time of it. I always fight this feeling and the proof is I have made it to this age (mid fifties) so this is a good thing. Thanks to my sons I have gotten this far. As in later years, it has been getting much harder, hence losing the battle and succumbing to three main goes at self-destruction.

I had been trying to fight off the feelings of depression all the previous day but I was having a very hard time this time round as it just kept coming at me, and I was feeling very overwhelmed. I am stuck in this moment forever and there is no escape. Claustrophobia has nothing on this for fear! I was looking for good things to try to counteract the feeling, but all that was coming to the fore was very black memories and the overwhelming feeling of being totally alone on the planet.

I think the feeling of being alone and of no use as if you are invisible is the hardest feeling to deal with. There seems to be a primal need to be part of something, a group, be it one person or a thousand. There is this need to "belong" somewhere in the scheme of things. My heart hurts for the elderly and the inept young men who have no one. The feeling of being alone has always been with me, but mostly only as a vague feeling. Then, it comes on so strong and it feels that I really am the only person here and everyone has left earth and gone somewhere else and forgotten me.

The despair was so overwhelming I had to try to stop it. The inner turmoil I experience when having a bad time and am unable to shake off is like having a major mudslide land on your head and having to walk around with it. The emotional turmoil and pain that goes on in my head for me to get to the stage of checking out was extreme. I realize now I cannot manage these depressions alone. I have tried and I know I need help to recover my self-worth and thus some appreciation of my role in life. When the outside world shrinks away, leaving just my demons with a stranglehold on me, I know another battle is about to start.

This is an educational tool if you like, in a way, that I will tell you how I felt and how my perceptions changed, as I got worse very quickly. I got to a level where I could not see my way back. It is better to understand the facts than imagine, guess, and have no understanding at all...

As far as I am concerned, it is a cancer of the mind. For

some people it lasts maybe a month or two, but for some it seems to last a lifetime. The analogy I would give is it is like Russian roulette: one bullet in a chamber of life. Is the depression deep enough to pull the trigger and will there be a bullet in the firing chamber?

If you can't imagine how tough it is so far, imagine this: a triathlon runner wins the race. He is exhausted to the extreme. Then he is told to get up and do it all again, straight away. No rest. No water. He has no reserves left; he has to get up and run again. He can't. He gives up there and then. He thinks the task is insurmountable. That is what it is like for me. I must keep going for my boys. I have nothing left but I have to keep getting up and continuing the journey for however long my body wants to torture me or until I die naturally.

So this particular day, the reserves were pretty low. I needed to crawl somewhere until it passed, but that is no good because it follows me. The next morning, after a restless night of fighting bad memories, I did not want to get out of bed to go to work. I didn't get out of bed to go to work. I couldn't. I didn't care anymore. I didn't care if I was sacked from my job at the bank. (Ironically, that was a contributor to my final demise, so it was a good thing to leave that environment.)

I lay in bed and just stared into space. I did not focus on anything in particular, as I was lost in a fog of confusion. I was numb. I could not function. This was when I knew I could not go on. And if the roof fell in, so be it. The thought of having one more day in this life made me want to throw up. I did eventually get out of bed and instead of my usual routine of staying in my room until washed, dressed and bed made, I become agitated and feel as though I am not part of the human race. I cannot remember what to do. The walls close in on me, which makes me feel as though I am suffocating. The house seems very quiet as though any external noises cannot penetrate the house. I just want to hide away from myself. It must be like a phobia really, a fear and a need to hide. My body is in a state of flight against a very big monster that wants to consume me. I can feel myself shrinking. I hate this shrinking feeling because inferiority, self-depreciation and a big sense of worthlessness comes with it.

I am getting smaller and smaller. I am consumed.

Out of desperation to escape the demons, I came up with an idea that I thought would make this emotional pain go away. I do not drink, as I have a low tolerance for alcohol. That seemed like the perfect answer. A quick reaction and then sleep. I went to the bottle store and purchased some alcohol of which I could tolerate the taste. To me, alcohol tastes very disgusting to the point where I feel like vomiting. Therefore, I had to get something that did the job of alcohol (like numbing the senses), but without the bad taste! I asked the shop assistant, a young boy (who incidentally looked like a ten-year-old) to show me the alcohol that did not taste like alcohol, but gave you the same effect, i.e. drunk! He did not think this a strange request as without missing a beat, he showed me some fancy-looking bottles that would meet my requirements. He said it tastes like milkshakes and was very popular with the young girls! Therefore, I purchased these bottles of "milkshakes." There were six in a pack, which was plenty for my low tolerance. Therefore, the sensible thing was to purchase them. So clutching this miracle cure for my demons, I was going to drown them in alcohol!

When I got home, I immediately opened one of these bottles to taste with a reservation that it would still taste like alcohol...but to my surprise, it really tasted like a milkshake. I was amazed and relieved. Now I could numb my brain and go to sleep. I expected it to be a little like rebooting the computer when it goes wrong! The caramel-flavored alcohol drink I had, which I hoped would put me to sleep until these demons left, only made me feel much worse and my demons got much bigger and stronger.

These alcohol milkshakes (as that is what they tasted of) are such a dangerous drink for young people who are not used to drinking (like me). It did not make me mellow, as I had hoped it would, because that is why I bought it in the first place. As a different remedy for the quick fix of depression...oh boy, it does not work!

I sat there waiting for the sleep to consume me, but I just got fuzzyheaded instead. Then the demons took over with a vengeance. All of the trauma I experienced just came and gave me a free showing, all over again. So as alcohol is a depressant anyway, I was in full-blown, down and slimy depression. At that point, there would not have been a person on the planet as worthless as myself. That is compliments of my negative, uncensored memories. I could not escape me. I was getting more and more lost in this horror show. There was no escape, no reprieve, and no mercy. The emotional pain was now overwhelming me to the point I could not think straight. I was losing touch with what was real and being sucked into this deep churning wave of depression with no way out. Seasickness is nothing compared to this. My mind was destroying me. I was nothing. I had nothing. This is what I was being bombarded with. If you ever saw "Clockwork Orange," there was a scene where Roddy McDowall had to keep looking at a movie with his eyes pinned open. He could not look away. It was shown to him repeatedly (horrible stuff, I think). Well that was going on in my head. Over and over. I was being bombarded with very negative stuff and personal attacks. A self-brainwashing, I suppose.

You cope with what life throws at you, don't you? Therefore, you cope. And you find ways to cope. And you have mental conversations with yourself to cope. And you can't possibly ask for help. And so you cope. And for me, over many years of coping, there had to be a consequence for this. And it came. It was as if the wind was sucked out of me all at once and I had nothing left to give. I had not one molecule of energy left to use. It was as if I had died already. I had hit rock bottom and there was nowhere else to go. (Up doesn't exist in the depressed mind at that level.) My picture of the waves crashing in shows where I was.

I am not sure what I should be doing right now. I should just go to sleep and hide from a monster that hounds me. Just until my anxiety goes away and the world stops bullying me. I think to myself that I have nothing to contribute to life, no value, a non-entity, so why stay and suffer. What is wrong with me? Why do I go into that black hole and am then consumed to such an extent that I do not know who I am. I can barely function physically, with everyday living when the depression descends. I feel I have hanging over my head the uncertainty of my ability to fight this off every time, and so feel I will lose the battle and if I lose the battle, so do my sons.

But I have to escape me. I pray that if there is a God and he created us, then I ask to be uncreated. I do not want to exist at all. The price to live is too high for me, in any form. I wanted to disappear into nothingness. I desperately want to stop trying to please, or be an emotional punch bag for others. I am not going to be good enough because I am never going to be cared about. I don't have the right ingredients — I know that now. No more mental torture to endure. It will soon be over. The alternative to living in a brutal world was death and silence. No more judgments and that was the only solution. I want it all to end. I do not know how to get back up again. The numbness, feeling alone and isolated, not measuring up — all these feelings are acute. It takes over body and soul. I feel it will go on forever, and I will start to believe hell would be preferable. This spilled over to the physical where I was having anxiety attacks often. But I was a walking contradiction. Externally I looked OK. I come across as jovial and this has been performed to perfection over the years. It is like a bandage hiding a big gash in your heart. I did not look like I was about to have a major crisis. I overcompensated for my internal turmoil. The reason for this was a fear of being found out that I can't cope anymore. I would be classed as subhuman if people saw my weakness in dealing with everyday life. I would be an outcast and ridiculed. Or talked about over drinks at a social gathering about how poor little Pat has lost the plot. What a pathetic creature she is.

It is silly to think anyone would want to do that, especially friends and family. But when you are in the grip of a meltdown, your thoughts and feelings become quite acute, blowing everything out of proportion and quite likely a little incorrect. Those old sayings are wise; making a mountain out of a molehill is apt for me. But just like people with phobias, i.e. frightened of going out their front door so they become a prisoner in their homes, this fear is real. They believe they are safe indoors so they must not go outside. So they stay captive and the jailer is their minds. Just like the jailer of my sanity is my mind also, for different reasons. I had to keep it together for a short time and then I could leave my tortured mind behind. This is where I started to go into myself and imagine no pain. No conflict. Especially "negative emotions," which in my case were dominating my every waking moment.

As I am writing this book, I feel fine and cannot imagine doing such a terrible thing. In fact, the thought of it frightens me very much. I love my life with my children and they are so wonderfully supportive. I have the two cutest dogs ever that keep me on my toes as well As two cats that rule the house and are wonderful. (You animal lovers out there know the warm feeling inside when you think of your pets; it is a very healing and loving feeling to own an animal you cherish, so you see, I don't want to die at all. I want to be there for my children.)

Sitting here, thinking about depression at the worst level, I cannot imagine what it is like, even though I have been down there...no, really. The terrible episode goes through a door and closes tight. So I cannot see the depth of despair I go down to. Women out there who have been through labour with the birth of a baby can understand that before the baby is born and the contractions are ripping you apart and you are crying out for a caesarean, it is the worst pain ever, but once the baby is born, the pain stops immediately. You cannot really imagine such pain now; you just know it was bad that is all. Then you go on to have another child and then suddenly remember, as the contractions get stronger and stronger, just how painful it is going to be as the memory that was locked away comes back to remind you! (Otherwise, if we remember, there would be no population. Of course, there are the lucky ones that have a very short labour and shed like peas with hardly any fuss.) But I did not want to acknowledge it. I wanted the last few minutes to go away but the power of the mind can control your emotions when you are vulnerable and so you have nothing extra to fight it with. But it had to be faced again. I was failing in the fight. I could not get out of the hole now; it was dark, slimy, and I could not fight it anymore.

I feel so inadequate; I just cannot pretend anymore. I am too broken emotionally. This, if you can imagine, is what I believed with all my being. It is not a "mood" or "self-pity"; it is profoundly more serious than minor "out of sorts moods." It is serious enough that I cannot bear to live anymore. This feeling takes over your whole being. This is a serious sickness. If you catch it early enough then it is handled and cured. If left too long, it becomes difficult to cure. This is very unhealthy thinking that should be stopped. If you do not understand any of this, great, but do not dismiss it as something as minor as a headache…it is a serious mental illness. If your child has it, he or she can die, and then you will get to know everything there is to know about the power of the mind and what it can do to you in the form of depression and deep anguish.

I was not born with mental illness; no one is, right? (There are some thoughts on hereditary, but I have not looked into it yet.) I personally think you survive this life OK even with all the battering you get. We all know sensitive people; they are lovely and in a way they find it harder to cope with life's challenges as they feel things deeply and may take on too much themselves.

You do not get to this state without the ingredients, i.e. abuse of all kinds, like emotional or physical abuse. Trauma in their life they have not dealt with, which reoccurs PUTS (Post-traumatic stress disorder). Hormonal changes, i.e. teenagers and menopausal women and men. Lost love, which is very painful at any age. Bullying at schools can and does cause depression in the child, resulting in suicide. This is a broad spectrum, but there are so many more pressures in today's world, hence the increase in suicides. Religious beliefs (suicide bombers, they believe strongly in their cause; they cannot see it is wrong what they are doing, they are killing themselves because that is what they believe they should do).

These emotions were overwhelming like humiliation, despair and feeling so inadequate as a person. I hide my shame and make people think I am OK with my life, which is a tough job to do — believe me. Especially when all I want to do is crawl under the nearest rock, parked car, dog turd, anything as long as I can't be seen by the judging mob with their look of superiority and contempt for a pathetic human specimen like me. This constant feeling of failure drove me down and down until I could not get back up again. I had no more energy to rise above this sense of worthlessness.

The feelings of despair consumed me and I couldn't escape. I curled up into a little ball on the floor; I want to be invisible and hide from this torture. I know I had no rational thinking by this time, just a desperate need to get away from this pain. This level of distress is almost a physical pain, which starts in my chest and radiates to my head and abdomen. I cannot stand it any longer; I need to do something to get away and to be free of it. No more depression, no more demons. No more having to push myself to function. No more anything. I am now cocooned in a layer of cotton wool as I have very little self-preservation left, as it has been knocked out of me over the years. I have no fear of death. I do not have the usual self-protective barrier of survival instincts at the moment. I am going through the motions of living for the sake of my children.

Ironically, I hope 99.99 percent of people do not understand what I am saying here. To do so could only mean that you have been here yourself. We cannot understand what it is like for someone who has lost a limb. We can only guess and that would be miles off the mark to comprehend emotionally what it is really like for them.

The alcohol did not do it.

All I can think of is sleep. I need sleep now. I have done my job on this planet. I can go now. I go to the medicine cupboard and haul out all the pills I can find. These pills are toxic when taken too many. I took what was there, about sixty. You can die from taking as little as twelve of these. They are a sure thing. When I had taken them all, I went looking for more, just in case they did not work. But I had cleaned out the house now.

I sat down on the couch and had a sense of relief come over me. I mentally did a checklist of where my will was and if my boys knew where it was. They knew our lawyers name that had a copy of the will so I felt OK about that. What was strange, I suppose, was when I took the pills and was waiting to die, I felt I was abut to leave prison and was waiting in anticipation.

I had no thought of writing to the boys at this stage. It did not occur to me to do so, even though I am very close to them. I was, I suppose, very focused on my exit and nothing else really entered my head. Just the realization that soon it will all be over for me.
I had not even thought about who would find me. Or who would feed my animals.
I noticed I had not shaved my legs! What a silly thing to

notice especially as a short time earlier I had tried to kill myself.

I was brought to the emergency room by the ambulance. What a humiliation. I did not want to go into the ambulance with them; I wanted to stay at home, but there were two police officers and two ambulance officers saying if I don't go with them I would have to be taken with them without my permission. I had visions of being handcuffed by these young boys who looked no older than my own sons did. The indignity of these kids seeing me at my most vulnerable. It is so strange that I can feel humiliation at the same time as I am waiting to die. Maybe my mind was reminding me of what I would not be missing!

Am I supposed to feel something more profound, like fear or anger or apathy, but not humiliation? It feels like they caught me in my underwear in the middle of the octagon! Very strange combination, really. To be able to understand how I was feeling at the time, the ambulance officer obliged me and gave me some paper and a pencil to write with. I was very agitated at the time but I wanted to record my feelings, as they were so raw. What happens to me after I come out of the big, slimy black hole is that I have a tendency to forget the emotional side of the experience quickly. It is as if a door shuts after I leave the black hole and does not allow me to remember how I was feeling at the time. I certainly can remember my actions, but not the emotions of what drives me to such extreme actions as taking an overdose. The emotions are not forthcoming once I get back to a more stable state of mind.

This is what I wrote as I was taken to the hospital by ambulance. (I automatically have a need to write when I am in a very dark place). It is in a way like a suicide note. I have to reach my family to let them know how I felt at the time of this episode, and to let them know "I know not what I do" at the time. This may seem bazaar, but writing this book may be the only way I can let my children know it is a disease and I could not fight off this current episode. It is a mind-numbing, debilitating decease. There are no choices open to you at the time. Your mind has been consumed by very negative, incorrect thinking. It can be all-consuming. For example, someone having a seizure cannot decide to stop it at that moment, they have to ride it through to the end. You cannot stop. It is a very hard-to-understand decease when you cannot see any "physical" illness. You have to try to understand what has happened to bring them to their knees in an overwhelming sense of failure and pain.

Maybe if I go to sleep, it will go away and I will be OK again. I am incapable of phoning anyone; my will is so diminished it would be like climbing a big mountain in extreme conditions to get to the top where a telephone may or may not be found! I feel trapped with these feelings to such an extent that there is no timeframe. It feels like these feelings will last for eternity. That is the most horrible feeling, the thought there is no way out of this. I feel like a five-year-old child stuck in the middle of a huge city like New York where no one knows me and I am just standing there, invisible. No one can see me; I am ignored as the people walk by. I do not know if there is a safe place for me. It feels like I am very alone.

Who will look after me? A minute feels like an eternity. What am I supposed to do? I do not know what to do. I think I should sleep this nightmare away now. I am incapable of responsibility for myself right now. What am I supposed to do? I am in a void that consumes me and will last forever unless I can get away from it. Sleeping is a good thing. I do not feel the pain there. If I do not have a plan in place for when I start to feel I am losing control of my emotions, I slide fast. I wanted to hide from the world and all it demands. To hide from my tortured mind, to escape the constant self-delusions that I know I have about myself but are so ingrained into my very soul, I cannot seem to escape them. So what is wrong with that?

I am so detached from this drama, I am not sure if I posses any kind of emotions at all — well not that I am looking. It is quite good not to feel sometimes. Therefore, this is not so bad. Therefore, I wait to die. It is only time now and soon I can sleep. I rationalize this by knowing I have brought the kids up to be good, confident young men and they are now grown up and independent. I think I have broken some promises but I'm not sure what they are now. Maybe I will remember later. I am no good. I think these pills will finally release me from my demons.

CHAPTER TEN

Well I am in the emergency department at the hospital with "guards." I thought it would be over by now, but it is not. I am still here and I miscalculated the amount of aspirin you need to take to end the pain. I am still stuck in A & E feeling like a hypochondriac.

It was supposed to have done the job effectively. I know what I felt at the time, as I am obsessive about writing down my feelings, which I have done for a number of years just to try to understand the deep chasm I fall into, and why and to survive repeatedly even though I did not want to be here.

When I conclude that the only way was suicide, and then I had a feeling of peace, a sense of having it over with consumed me. It was like a magic pill, it would cure all my pain.

What was real to me was that the outside world did not exist at this point. It was just my demons and me. You do not think, oh poor boys will be without their mother. No, I thought logically and not emotionally. The emotional side of me went into liquidation, I think. I became just an analytical robot that had a job to do. I mentally went through what insurance policies I had. This in order, I was ready for my journey to exodus. I also thought it was OK because my children are grown men now and do not need me. Very rational and orderly thinking. So as you can see, it is not a normal way to be. I was going down the "green mile" in a sense and there were no emotions. Just a job to finish. In a bazaar way, it was like being organized and ready to go on a long holiday. Moreover, the mindset is focused on this journey; I could function as if nothing at all is wrong in the world if anyone turned up at that moment. They would not have a clue as to what I was about to do. I do not know where this comes from, and how the mind can organize its self-destruction so rationally, but it did. Maybe the word is temporary insanity.

 Our emotions are taken out of the equation for this journey; only the rational thinking is present so the effect on family and friends does not come into it at all. Not because we do not care; on the contrary, we do, very much. However, it is more like a personal journey. It would be like wondering how your family is going to cope if you go on holiday; well you do not think that — you're too busy thinking of your journey.

When I am having a bad time of it, I write in my journal exactly how I am feeling so that I can try to understand what is going on and if there is anything triggering these episodes of depression. What I do find interesting is that my handwriting changes as I go down the slippery slop. Usually it is adultish, neat and an italic style. But when I go down, it changes to childish handwriting. When I am at the bottom.

I did a painting of how I felt a few years ago. I feel as if I'm in a time warp as I haven't exorcised that feeling yet. It is still there just as strong as it was all those years ago.

This is what takes over my thinking and emotions. In addition, I believe the negative crap that consumes my mind, body and soul. Like being consumed by an evil spirit..., that is a bit melodramatic, but you get the picture.

Obviously I didn't die as I am still here writing these five hours later with a short break as I keep puking up whatever my body decided it could do without! I didn't need a stomach pump, as my body ruled against my wishes to die and ejected this crap quite efficiently all by itself and with a hint of humiliation thrown in for good measure!

What do I feel about the fact I could have died tonight. NOTHING. Maybe at a pinch, apathy, a sense of failure. Lost. I can't cry because that is so far up the ladder; it is near happiness.

I'm definitely not looking forward to the inevitable onslaught of interrogation from family/psychiatrists and psychologist, and whoever else. I guess it is to be expected to feel lethargic considering I have dosed up on a lot of drugs and alcohol. I wish I could hide in a hole and be forgotten. I have nothing more to contribute to this world and if there is anything, it is minor anyway.

I have been transferred to EPS (emergency psychiatric services). Whilst waiting for the doctor, my defunked system continues to house clean, so I rushed for the nearest waste paper bin and started puking my guts up, and at the same time my butt decided to join in the "lets humiliate pat fiasco" and release some pressure also. Oh the indignity of it all, so I was puking and tooting at the same time. Retrospectively, it was quite funny for me to disgrace myself in such a way!

Taking a huge overdose and how I felt waiting to die. Then how I felt when it didn't happen as it should, which is what I desperately wanted at the time? I wanted to die. I wrote my thoughts at the time while waiting for my system to shutdown. Therefore, I did what was necessary to die. I am obsessive about writing, so I even wrote as I was going through the process so maybe someone out there could understand what goes through the mind of someone prior to committing suicide thus I scribbled on pieces of paper constantly as my mood changed. Even when I was dragged into the hospital. They gave me more paper at the emergency department, but I guess they thought I was wacko anyway so obliged, which was nice...strange behavior but necessary, I feel. I knew I would not remember if I survived this and then how can I make the boys understand how I felt then. And if I did not survive, my sons can read what I felt throughout that process. The psychiatrist took a copy for his files. I see it as a peephole into this bazaar behaviour.

I remember I did not want anyone to know about my problems. I wanted to pretend I had not a care in the world. I thought that if people knew about me battling depression (caused by my problems) then I would seem weak and useless; therefore, ashamed. In addition, part of the problem was I would have to betray and expose, and so doing would feel I was the traitor, so would feel even worse! (A no-win situation.) So I am silent, just like many other people who carry burdens and then get depression because of it.

The "doctor" has come to see us. Immediately I had my hackles up. I felt defenseless against this "authority." I felt like a child and was going to be punished and belittled by him. These are the kind of emotions you deal with when you're down in the pits. The reality is very different, but I did not know that, of course. I was in the middle of my episode. Your emotions are not your friend when you're down there, which makes the feelings exponentially stronger.

The psychiatrist comes into the room and sits in the chair opposite me — well he sort of lounges in the chair really; I wonder if that was to try to be "cool" or just lazyassed because he could not be bothered to sit up and talk to me. I was feeling very prickly towards him, and he had not opened his mouth yet. It is amazing how you can size someone up in a second when you're full of drugs and totally neurotic at the time, but are convinced of your diagnosis of the man.

The way he talks to me I found to be very condescending and I told him so. My state of mind, I am sure, is contributing in a big way to the way I see this person. However, at the time, I felt like punching him in that smirking, priggish, irritating face of his. (I am sure it is not paranoia on my part...!)

He looks like a learned textbook kid, someone who has never ever gone through depression to any degree in his entire — smug fucking life. He almost looks bored, he is wearing this expression on his face that reads, yeah, yeah, yeah, whatever, let's get you moved on, so I can go back to my PlayStation game. (F*****g dim whit) now this is how I felt at that time. I don't know where the anger came from but I had it there, boiling over. Funny how I never get angry when I am OK. I am basically very laid back and placid.

I am sure in the light of day he is quite a nice person and is not as I portray him but when you are totally off your head, a cute cuddly rabbit could look like a rabid dog!

What I was feeling at the time was acute agitation. Again, I don't know why I feel like this, it is not normal in my life other than when I am like this. Moreover, I had nowhere to dump it other than in his face, poor sod. My emotions went from a state of apathy to agitation and if it was to be rated from one to ten, it would be off the scale. (Hmmm, talk about a roller coaster ride, this is far scarier.) I feel like a caged lion; I can't escape them or my feelings, or me. It sucks.

Anyway, as we sat opposite each other I felt we were covertly clashing. If you could burn someone with your eyes, he would have a hole burned in his head and likewise for me too as I saw it. (It is amazing what you assume when you are so psychotic.)

I feel as if I'm on trial and he is the prosecutor. I can't remember what he said to me, but obviously not intelligent enough for me to warrant a mention of his dialog. If I remembered, it would be something like this. Who is the Prime Minster? Who is Moby Dick? He is now talking to my son (it is about one am and my poor son has had to watch his mother go through the dramas of the day to this incarceration by the authorities that be!) I have no idea how he must be feeling, He is being so gentle and supportive of me in this awful situation, but I am too far removed from the real me to take anything in on an emotional level that is normal. (It's just paranoia now.)

I look over to where my son is standing and he looks very tired, as it is very late and we both have not eaten since lunchtime and are both susceptible to low blood sugar and get the shakes and cannot think straight. He has been on this emotional roller coaster for many hours now, especially with knowing your mother tried to kill herself. I can't imagine what he must be feeling now.

I feel very groggy and lightheaded, but continue to dry wretch now. Boy is my body rebelling against the abuse it got!

I am fuzzyheaded but I feel I am coming out of my deep slimy hole of depression. I am feeling a little more in control of my feelings now. The monster is going back into the black slimy hole from whence it came. Nevertheless, that does not let me off the hook. I still have to address this current attempt with my family and the medical professionals. They are still going to lock me up in a secure ward "for my own protection." I still feel very vulnerable and insecure about myself.

When this black slimy fog consumes me, I cannot see anything — and I don't mean blind physically, just mentally. I cannot feel anything other than a desperate, overwhelming pain inside of me. It consumes me. Some of the feelings I try to identify are feelings of being inadequate, insignificant and alone. It is as if my brain is working against me and my survival instincts are diminished. The nearest I can get with the description of my mental illness is it is like a cancer. It consumes you with feelings of acute emotional pain and if you do not find a cure or remission, your prognosis is grim. You can only take so much of this abuse of the self.

Think of dominos in a long trail where if you knock one down the lot goes. Well in a way, the trigger that causes the downward spiral is like that. I get one bad reminder of past pain that I have not dealt with, then wham, the first domino crashes. The reaction is so fast it is hard to holt it. Then there I go, head first into the slime. It is an automatic chain reaction in my brain. If you were burned by fire, you will always have a respect for it in the future and not go near it otherwise you will be burned again. Well the body has automatic responses, both good and bad. Mine is a bad response that I can't seem to stop when it is triggered.

If this sounds melodramatic, well good, it is the nearest I can get to conveying the debilitating effect depression can and does have on people with this hideous mental cancer that eats you alive. Well, my son has talked with the doctor for about half an hour now, while I continue going through the motions of puking. I didn't know you can do muscle exercises this way because my tummy muscles really hurt now. (I'll find the correct name for the tummy muscles later, OK.)Now as I expected, the doctor has decided it is better to have me go to the ward overnight and then be assessed fully tomorrow, which is today because it is two am.

Also, it was suggested my son get some sleep, as it has been a tough day for him. He would not sleep if I were at his house because he would be too worried about what I might do. So sensible decision, my boy needs his sleep. I don't want him worrying all night about me. He shouldn't have to go through this stuff. But again, there should not be mental illness. But there is. So in a dazed surreal way, I said goodnight to my son and he promised to be at the hospital early the next day. I said he didn't have to come early but knowing my son, he did anyway. I am a very lucky mother, and I know it. So can you imagine what it must feel like when you come out of the depression to the chaos I created and cause such grief to my sons, I certainly need a lot of therapy, even if it is for this part.

I am supposed to be a mother who would protect and never let anything hurt my boys. But I hurt my boys in a bad way. I was taken to the psychiatric hospital secure ward. This is where you are locked up. Now that sounds bad, but it is obviously in the interest of the patients to keep them safe while they arrange for you to be seen by a specialist in this field, in this case a psychiatrist. I think they are to be commended for doing this type of job. Not only are they walking on eggshells (definitely in my case), they know they must not inflame the situation any further for the patient. That is dealing with some very bad issues of various kinds and perhaps trying to find a big bridge to jump off.

The next day my son collected me from the psychiatric ward and took me to his house to stay with him and his wife, which he found emotionally very hard, seeing his mum incarcerated in a secure unit where the doors are locked so you cannot get out by yourself and you have no rights as regards to leaving on your own free will. (A suicide attempt takes those rights away as you are deemed a danger to yourself.)

He sat me down and said mum, if you commit suicide, it would be like handing my brother and me your depression. We would suffer greatly because of your actions, and I personally would not want to have children if you were not here to be a part of our lives. That would be the consequences of your actions. I would like you to sit down and do a painting for me, showing you have your boy's future in your hands. So you can see I have lovely boys who really care and love me. But I still tried to kill myself. I am so grieved to think I have caused my family such anxiety and pain when I tried to kill myself. Sadly, for them, this was not the first time I tried. But suicidal depression makes a mockery of such things as loving families, good friends, great lifestyle, etc. — you could have all this and still succumb to depression and suicide because it can be totally consuming as in my case. I want my children to understand how very incapable I was of making rational decisions at that time. (The psychologist/psychiatrists call it an episode.) I thought about what my son said and I could visualise how I was coping at that moment and painted this picture, which is at the back of the book with sample explanations. I am only frightened that I would succumb when I am OK again and realise how close I came to death. But by the powers that be, I hope to live out my life naturally and die when my time is up, and not before. I want to make my sons proud of me for fighting it and never ever giving up, until the monster is defeated. And I shall have won the biggest battle of my life.

The picture I painted, which is at the end of the book, is of me standing in a pit of burning coals that represent my depression, which is hell and the only thing keeping me from crashing and burning is my children. The butterflies symbolise my sons needing their mum. In addition, at all costs, they must not be burned by the fires of hell (depression) and it is up to me to hold on and keep them; the only way I could show what has kept me going and pushing on all these years. I know my children will go forward in life and give love and support to their own children, especially knowing how very important it is to feel wanted and loved. (They know my history and what effect it has on me emotionally to have none of this.) I guess once the setting is set, you have to use the tools you are given in life to survive; the main thing is knowing that you are a worthwhile person who is wanted and loved. That I am sure is my foundation to build on, to grow up strong and healthy emotionally with a sense of who you are and where you belong in the scheme of things.

It is a tough playground if you have no self-worth.

CHAPTER ELEVEN

A young person says, starting puberty allows him to experience what women experience when they go through menopause; that is, mood swings influenced by hormones. The hormones are adjusting and increasing or decreasing the quantities the body needs. Main timeframes are puberty, pregnancy and menopause. This is not including illnesses such as thyroid problems, etc. The body is an amazing machine if you consider there is so much to the body that we are still learning about and discovering (especially the brain).

Women know the change of life can be very depressing and not pleasant in the least. (This is regarding women who do not sail through menopause as others do.) The hormones certainly let you know they are downsizing or upsizing! I have been through menopause, and for me I did not really notice the mood swings as I was in a world of mood swings anyway. And now all I have to show for it is a beard and beer belly!

But seriously, it can be very disruptive to the smooth running of the home when patience goes out the door along with that youth who is changing also. What a combination...

Note to mothers going through the change and who have teenagers: forget diet; indulge in some nice goodies or pampering of some kind and a good book or two and wait it out. You only have a couple of years or so. That is not so bad. But I warn you, you may need to go on a diet again when it is all over. Jenny Craig will love you.

Or better still, go on holiday until it is safe to come

home; by then the youth will become the lovely normal "trainee" adult you once knew! Well, you can only hope or go join a foreign legion — life would be much easier there, and I am sure. Only kidding...by the way, this includes fathers. It can be as tough for you too. Imagine a wife and child going through changes and the prerequisite for them is to dump their sense of humour in the bin as not needed for a couple years. So for fathers and husbands, buy a joke book and make yourself laugh otherwise you go to the foreign legion too. Parents and guardians out there who are laughing at the thought of a teenager going through puberty "silently" may be stretching the imagination a bit, as they can be very vocal, as you know. But seriously, it is a very vulnerable age for them. I am not digressing: teenagers are a whole bag of contradictions in themselves. Do not underestimate how tough it is for them physiologically because it affects how they function emotionally...

As you know, puberty is changing of the body also and can be a tough time for some. The hormones are talking. Young people go through this with hardly a blemish on their face and/or with a good disposition, and some go through it with the explosion of frustration, anger, sulky duos, and to top it off their once smooth skin turns into acne almost overnight. Suddenly they have to deal with all sorts of issues that take them out of the child category forever and dump them in what I would call all no-mans land. They are neither a child nor an adult in the sense of the word...

They have to know how to deal with their own particular problem on their own if they do not talk to anyone about it. I remember going through a huge self-pity phase when I was about fifteen years old. My poor friend had many ear bashings from my constant moaning about all and nothing. I do not remember her doing the same; she was easy going as I remember. But again, she probably did not get a word in with me.

We do not want to walk in someone else's footsteps, as our own are tough enough at times. But generally, we can try to have more understanding and compassion for others in all lifestyles. We still feel pain the same. We are mothers and fathers, brothers, sisters in all cultures, creeds and races. We have to struggle on with our grief wherever we are born in the world. So, what I am saying is, there is more to the people who commit suicide. They were unable to deal with their problem or talk to someone because quite likely they felt unable to do so. You cannot underestimate the force of our emotions, which can hold you back from getting help. There is a checkout point in us all. Most of you would never reach it or comprehend how others can. It had gotten beyond normal emotions in a way. I know the feeling well. You isolate yourself. You do not want to talk. In a way, if you do not talk, it does not exist.

It is like trying to have a deep meaningful conversation with your teenager when they barely talk to you, and if they did talk it would be that one syllable grunting noise that they are so good at; at that stage only their friends can understand them. It is almost impossible to get anything comprehensible out of them (special teenage language). I am not making fun of teenagers but I do remember when my boys were teenagers, I could not have a conversation with them until I think they were around twenty years old. Suddenly they talked normally, used many more syllables, and complete sentences. A very depressed person finds it just as hard to vocalise their pain to anyone. A very lonely road is traveled to commit suicide. They are beyond normal grief or pain. If you saw me just before I took an overdose of many certain drugs that guarantee destruction of the liver and other organs to a slow death, I looked well balanced and fine. I could have a conversation, but it would be robotic or going through the motions of politeness. Then I'd go home and organise my demise.

Negative thinking is distorted thinking and denies oneself of positive feelings. Well, I know this logically and emotionally but the rules change when you succumb to mood change, which is when the fight begins in earnest.

This is how complex the body is. For a start, it takes years for medical students to study the complexities of the human body. When you think about it, to study the body is a huge undertaking. Even for a genius let alone your average high-grade student. Therefore, the body has been divided into sections (i.e. blood is studied by haemo dudes; bones are studied by skeleton dudes; a neuropathologist studies your nerves, your muscles are studied by mycologist hormones by a horny dude. Y dudes, the heart is studied by a cardiologist. You see what I mean). Our bodies are taken for granted and we abuse it and still expect it to function (i.e. alcohol, smoking, poor diet, drugs). This, of course, is stated simply as each body part that is studied interconnects with the next section, so I guess they need to know something of everything in the body. But specialise in the one area of the body.

However, the aim is in letting people know there really is help out there. Do not hide the problem; it can become all consuming to the point of driving you down to hell. The weapon as doctors, psychologists, and psychiatrists know is first talk, then together work from there, depending on your problem. However, this service is not utilised enough due to a number of reasons, so action does not take place and hence a high suicide rate in the western world.

CHAPTER TWELVE

I know what I am talking about regarding suicide as I have been down that road and am still recovering. In addition, I realised how little people know of the mechanics of mental illness.

From the dictionary:

MENTAL: relating to the mind; found in; occurring in the mind. Mental stimulation.

ILLNESS: a disease, (sickness; an impaired condition; an unsound or corrupt condition) or indisposition.

So the definition in this case for mental illness is an impaired condition occurring in the mind. This is what I would like you to understand when reading this book. They had an undiagnosed illness. Someone with cancer of the body dies; you would never call them selfish for dying, would you? They had an illness of the body. Suicidal people have an illness of the mind. We have misconceptions about why someone has taken his or her life. If there is no answer with say a suicide note, then there is only speculation. And you know what we are like when we speculate. Usually we are way off the mark. We should not judge them, as they have judged themselves. People need educating and to get a better understanding of mental health. Because let's face it, it affects us all, at some stage, whether it be friends, relatives or even yourself. And as the saying goes, to be for warned, is to be forearmed. (This answer came up most often when asked what they thought of people who kill themselves.) This is so not correct. It is like saying a cancer patient is selfish for dying! They were both ill, one bodily and one mentally. The body was attacked and destroyed by cancer cells. The mind destroyed the body with mental cancer.

The Invisible Stalker

We underestimate the power of the mind. It can make you walk on hot coals without feeling the heat. It can make you go into a trance and do what the hypnotist commands. People put meat skewers in their bodies and hang themselves up to show what they can do. Soldiers of good standing and are generally nice people go out and gun down and kill innocent women, children and the elderly, who are completely defenseless.

These ordinary people live in little villages in the middle of nowhere. They have done nothing to threaten the soldiers. They do not have weapons, or anything that could be seen as a threat. But the soldiers were told to kill the villagers. This could be your son doing this atrocity. You could not imagine it, could you? But he along with his regiment was told to do it. So they did.

The mind can make you do many things you think your incapable of doing, even killing yourself for that matter, we call it suicide. Never underestimate the power of your mind and the hold it can have over you..

Nevertheless, if you asked the soldier if he could gun down the people who are defenseless, he would probably say "hell no." But he does because his superior officers ordered the troops to carry out the action plan to take over the village. Sadly, this scenario is a fact of war (Vietnam. There's gruesome evidence in the war museums there). So you see, there are many examples of how powerful the mind is to such an extent, it can do things you would never ever imagine you could do.

Imagine what family and friends feel when this happens to someone who "has everything" (I'm talking on the top end of the spectrum of people and what they have in life, never mind the poor souls who are homeless and have no one and doped up or drunk every day/night to keep out the misery and numb the mind for just a little while. In addition, as winter is coming and they are homeless and contemptuous nobodies as far as society is concerned...this is the other end of the scale. Suicide does not discriminate!

The gauge to misunderstanding this mental illness for me is people saying random things like they died because they were selfish and didn't think of their families or he or she didn't talk to me, etc. some people with this illness only get diagnosed after trying to kill themselves. Then they get the help they need to recover fully. This can be a short road; maybe short courses of medication to help you while you are working through your problems with the professional community who have many resources to help on the road to recovery. Of course, as you may know, I am talking from experience. I had to go into a world of wonderful people who care and are dedicated to your recovery. I was amazed once I could appreciate the dedication they had for helping me to recover.

CHAPTER THIRTEEN

When I look at my sons, I feel as proud as only a parent knows and very blessed to know they are my children. They are both very kind, considerate young men and we have a close relationship.

So why would I want to kill myself and totally devastate them and probably scar them emotionally for life? Maybe it is because I am so selfish; I only care about me. Alternatively, I am attention seeking. Or maybe I do not love them. Or I have a fixation on death and want to see what it is like. (That last comment was from a young man who nearly shot himself, but luckily did not, and said he wanted to know what it would be like!)

These people have given me permission to mention their stories. There were many more, sadly a few very young people amongst them, but I just wanted to share these with you and to make you aware there are far too many of these tragedies for the victim and the kin. Everyone hurts; no one escapes this kind of thing. There has to be more we can do to recognise, take action and avert this from happening too often in all societies. There is a reason, we just need to find it and cure it. Again, I still think it is a mental cancer that becomes unbearable, but is invisible to society and takes its toll.

There is not enough said about this sort of tragedy and most of the time it is swept under the carpet by society as a whole due to the enormity of the problem. There are people as young as ten years old and as old as eighty plus years (not with a terminal illness and euthanasia that has nothing to do with this sort of suicide).

A few of the stories are very similar and so it seems more common than we realise. I have not looked up the statistics, as it is too depressing to imagine all those people out there that have to deal with the loss of someone to this heinous and not very well-documented mental decease. It is not a cry for help; it has gone far beyond that because they have died. They took the action that would make sure they did it once only. With a cry for help, where they take an overdose, they tell someone, and then get help. They need to be taken very seriously too, as in the end, if the problem still overwhelms them and they are not having help dealing with it or it gets worse, then they may give up too. As it is so silent and there seems to be no warning, it is very hard to prevent, unless you know what you are looking for. Evan a qualified practitioner can find it hard to recognise and they are trained to do such things.

There seems to be a stigma attached to the word and act of "suicide." Stemming from religious beliefs and the power of this belief still torments the grieving person today and may continue to do so until we can really analyze the power depression can have over someone to the extent they cannot take it any more and kill themselves. When you are down there, purgatory seems like a haven for the broken spirit. For the religious folk, it must be especially painful if they are thinking their loved one has gone to purgatory or some such place and is not "with their God."

These people have lost their family member and they have the added grief of thinking the person will not get to salvation. Then they question themselves and wonder where they went wrong in bringing their child up in their faith and making sure that they know suicide is a sin against their god. I have no affiliation with any church, but as a young person, I did the rounds of the religious faiths, looking for my own salvation from life's burdens, but found only empty words and rituals, which I found irrelevant. Other people found great solace in their religion, which is good, as sometimes we need all the help we can get on our journey through life. I go it alone, as I cannot lose what I have not found in a heavenly body, but I envy those who have found faith in a higher being.

I think the thing that stood out about the people I talked to is that none had counseling to help them get to understand the myriad of emotions they are experiencing. By doing that alone it can help them move forward enough to bear the pain of the loss.

The most common question is why. This is the most frustrating for them and as one woman said, if she knew why she could start to come to terms with it and maybe try to understand. If only they could have a minute with them again to make it all better as only a terrible void is left.

CHAPTER FOURTEEN

These are examples of the sort of comments people make when they do not understand the illness. It is an illness...this illness is invisible until the signs and symptoms show up by way of change in behavior, for instance (i.e. not sleeping, eating too much, not eating, lethargy, cry for no reason or for the slightest thing, and cannot get motivated at all). Self-appearance and personal hygiene can slip. It is too much of an effort to dress, wash and comb your hair, which starts the neglect of oneself. Getting angry at the smallest thing. Being anxious all the time. Even hysteria for no reason. Isolating yourself when normally you are outgoing. There are some signs that show up as a red flag. If you consider that depression can ultimately kill, early signs are giving you warning before it escalates. That it will just go away without any medical intervention, well that would be great. But the ones that ignore it, and it does not go away, they end up dead! Is this brutal enough for you? I want it to be because some of our youngsters are not coping with whatever it is that has triggered their depression, and they end up killing themselves. People need to be educated in getting some understanding of this killer decease. You probably know someone who has died from suicide. It is a killer and then it does not stop there, it goes on to destroy families by unbearable grief. So you see, it does not just affect that person who died — it affects all of us. Just like if he had a broken limb, you would go see someone to get it fixed. And most importantly without any fear of retribution from peers.

For people who recognise this saying, "father, forgive them for they know not what they do," is so true in this respect, even though we think we know what we are doing. Please forgive our transgression into momentary insanity.

The reason why I got suicidal (which is a mental illness) is not the issue or even relevant in this book. Let me expand on that. To get to the same place, that is, to want to take our own lives, comes from very many sources to this pivotal point (i.e. abuse, sodomy, rape, guilt, emotional and physical abuse). Loneliness, as in the aged or social outcast. Heartbroken from lost love. Teenagers who suffer hormonal imbalance and thus suffer mood swings to excess. Bullying. Bankruptcy. The list is infinite. However, the point is what happens to you to make you take that final step to end it all in suicide? Were there any calculated actions like months or weeks or even days before? Do you wake up one day and decide next Wednesday you're going to kill yourself and tough on the rest of the world. Do you think you are going on a holiday and are flippant about knowing you are going to die?

I do not know, but for myself, I can answer questions that would need to be told to my loved ones if given the chance.

Sometimes this deliberate act can make it hard to move forward for the bereaved, as they have no conclusive answers as to why. They can feel guilt, anger, confusion, despair, and great sadness. On top of this, they do not know where to turn for answers. Is this the sort of legacy I would have left to my children...?

When I start to feel down, I write in my journal about my feelings at the time, mainly to try to make sense of them later, when I am more levelheaded. Over the years, I have noticed a consistency of perceived thoughts at the time of having a depressive episode. I did not think for one moment that the doctors could help me at all. Oh no, sir! I thought they were quacks who had no idea about how I was feeling. How can they — they did not live my life. They did not experience or understand what I feel. I expected them to just give me some pills and send me home.

How very wrong I was.

My psychologist has worked very hard with me to dispel my delusions about myself with huge improvements and much much less fear being carried on my shoulders. If I were never to go back into society, I would no doubt handle the negative side of me without too much of a fight. Yes, it is fights I have with myself. Or should I say my mind. You know what I mean, when the negative thoughts invade your thinking and you cannot look at something with a positive spin on it. I know that is normal to some extent and OK as long as it doesn't drag you down beyond normal thinking.

However, as life is not so simple, I have to be part of society and all the ups and downs, which is where I am most vulnerable.

From my waking hour, I am fighting with the need to hide from the world. There is little let up of this feeling and to help me get through a day, I pretend I am invisible to people, which gives me a small sense of security.

My outward package that people see is this bubbly but ditzy girl and I am fine with that, thanks you very much. I think this persona doesn't encourage too much scrutiny as I just look the ditzy type and warrant no further investigation from anyone.

The Invisible Stalker

I do not usually have eye contact with anyone because I do not want to be challenged on anything real or imagined. No contact, no stress. No problems. No dark place to fall into.

If somehow when you are going to kill yourself, the mind lets in the emotional side and you think of the consequences to your kin, then maybe many suicides would not have occurred, my attempts included. However, when it seems like it will last forever and is unbearable, so the bullet seems the only option. One of the things people constantly say is why didn't they come to me? Well, from my experience, when you are in a full-blown "had enough," you don't want to talk to anyone. You just do not. The focus is very strong on that silver bullet. It is saying to you, yes, your trouble (imagined or real) is going to be over forever. It is almost hypnotic. This is when you seek out isolation. The focus is absolute. Nothing gets in, and in a way, it is like sleepwalking. There are no rational feelings getting through, only the need to end it. I know my perceptions reverse when I am OK to when I am suicidal. I think I am rational when I am depressed but in fact I am thinking very dangerous thoughts regarding my value to 'society' and decide I am not needed here, so want to leave, and think I am being very rational and calm about it. It is as if I am planning a holiday; I think it through, make sure I have what I need, and then leave. When I feel I am going down into the slimy pit, I always imagine someone holding me and keeping me safe as if I was a newborn baby, and they would shield me no matter what because they think I am worth it.

A friend wrote a poem for me when he heard that I tried to "do myself in," and it went like this...

The tragedy of checking out
Are those you leave behind?
Will never know exactly what
Went on inside your mind.

They only know the love they gave
Was not enough to keep
Them ever present in your heart
Now they can never sleep.

It's guilt they feel for failing you
And just not being there
To help you when you needed help
In addition, show you that they care...

A well-meaning friend gave this poem to me...but sadly, as is the norm, he does not understand where I was at the time of the botched attempt of mine.

He also wrote this and said it may help. I was in the psychiatric ward at the time, due to falling head first into the slimy pit, putting it mildly! When he gave me this poem, he said that when I read the words, I must imagine and visualise each line as I read on...it is almost meditative.

Robert Free calls it somewhere.

Somewhere there's a rainbow
With its pot of gold
Somewhere there's a secret
Waiting to be told

Somewhere there's a shelter
To keep you from the storm
Somewhere there's a fire
To keep you safe and warm

The Invisible Stalker

Somewhere there's a candle
To give you hope and light
Somewhere there's a sunrise
To make the darkness bright

Somewhere birds are singing
Breezes softly blow
Flower buds are opening up
And putting on a show

Can you see their colours?
Can you smell their scent?
On every bloom the honey bee
Is full of good intent

Somewhere kids are laughing
Running, playing games
Somewhere there are paintings
Bigger than their frames

Somewhere there are wispy clouds
On bright blue sunny skies
Somewhere there are symphonies
That makes you close your eyes

Somewhere there are singers
Reveling in songs
Somewhere there are poets
Righting all the wrongs

Somewhere there are lovers
Walking hand in hand
Somewhere there are lapping waves
That gently kisses the sand

Somewhere there's a feathered bed

Patricia Reid

For you to snuggle in
Somewhere there's a handsome man
With a reassuring grin

Somewhere there's a present
Tied up with a bow
A letter in the letterbox
From someone that you know

Somewhere there are dresses
Stitched with your fair hand
And jars of pickled chutney
The best in all the land

Somewhere there are puppy dogs
And kittens lost in play
Somewhere there are swallow nests
Made of mud and clay

Somewhere there are three white ducks
Bathing in the sun
On the beach a panting dog
That wants to run and run

Somewhere thatched-roof cottages
Line leafy country lanes
Where early morning foxes
Avoid the summer rains

Somewhere there are raindrops
That trickles down your back
Somewhere an alpine flower
Is bursting through a crack

Somewhere there are forest streams
Lakes of azure blue
Mountainsides of virgin snow

The Invisible Stalker

Leaves with drops of dew

Meadows filled with little lambs
That leaps and prances with glee
Somewhere there's an albatross
Soaring out to sea

Somewhere leaves are rustling
Shimmering the trees
Somewhere there's a skylark
High up in the breeze

Somewhere yachts are sailing
Somehow they seem to cope
Even when there is no wind
Their sails are filled with hope

Somewhere there are all these things
And all these things are true
For if, you have imagined them
They're all inside of you

You are where the somewhere is
You are all these things
Draw your strength from what you are
The joy that being brings

You are all you need to be
You're all of the above
Know that people love you
And know that you can love

It was beautiful, simple and above all, I could see these things in my mind's eye and for that moment in time, I was in the poem, in another dimension, where I was able to be. With no torment. Just like the pictures I paint, I lose myself in them.

Patricia Reid

A poem of defiance

Big black hole here I come
Big black hole, cold and numb
You do not scare me because I shake my bum
And I say, pooh pooh to you

I can smile because I'm free
And my heart is full of glee
I laugh ha ha and I laugh hee hee
And I say pooh pooh to you

I've got better things to do
Than entertain the likes of you
I've seen better things
On the bottom of my shoe
So I say pooh pooh to you

I know I'll be happy soon
When I sing this happy tune
And I'll have sex in the afternoon
If I want so pooh pooh to you

Robert Free the poet

Recovering From Suicide Loss

By Lorraine A. Winsey, RN, Patient Care Manager Inpatient Psychiatric Services

Recovery means to regain, to get back to or to restore. It is a process of learning to deal with each day's challenges. In regard to suicide loss, a significant lessening of most of the emotions that you are feeling right now marks recovery. Suicide loss makes you vulnerable to a wide range of problems. Depression and severe anxiety reactions can occur. Complicated grief reactions can occur. Worst of all, suicidality can occur.

Suicide loss is the most horrible loss that anyone can suffer. You may feel betrayed, angry, out of control, disoriented and hurt. You may feel that the one you lost has let you down by leaving you behind to mourn. You may feel anger that your loved one never gave you the chance to help. You may feel guilt or responsibility because you feel you should have or could have done something to prevent this. You have lost your emotional bearings and you can find nothing in your past experience to help you cope.

Every suicide is different and the circumstances leading up to it are always unique to the individual involved. However, many studies of suicide suggest that it comes about because of intense psychological pain and extreme feelings of hopelessness on the part of the individual taking his or her life. Many of those suffering depression may make some effort to hide it. This is especially the case with male teenagers and men. Some may not have realized that they were suffering from depression. Others, if they asked for help, felt they would appear weak and would incur shame or stigma.

Patricia Reid

Feeling suicidal is a tremendous psychological burden that may distance those bearing it from those who care about them. Most suicidal individuals do not really want to die. They just want to end the pain and hopelessness. Many of those who complete suicide struggle with this ambivalence to the end. It is becoming clear that suicide is strongly related to changes in the brain and to chemical imbalances in the body. These factors may override the individual's ability to reach out.

Suicide is not predictable. To some degree it can be determined that someone may be at risk of completing suicide. However, there is no way to definitely project it or when a particular individual may complete suicide.

Suicide loss does follow a pattern. There doesn't seem to be a standard grieving process that we all go through. It is different for each of us in terms of what or when things happen. There does seem to be some phases that we each experience. There is the dissonance phase. This is the initial period after the loss and you can feel panic, blame and incrimination. This may be followed by the debilitation phase which can make you feel a loss of control over your life, a sense of powerlessness. Eventually you rebound and the acute nature of your grief subsides and you are in the desensitization phase. You are still vulnerable to relapses at this phase. And finally there is the differentiation phase. You are not better or stronger; you are just "different." You can function better and, except for that residual sense of loss that will always be with you, you feel normal again. These phases can takes months or years.

You should contact your health care provider as soon as possible after your loss. Working through your grief in a group setting with other people that understand your pain can be therapeutic and help you through your tragedy.

Two good places to visit on the internet for information on suicide:

- American Foundation for the Prevention of Suicide (www.afsp.org)

- American Association of Suicidology (www.suicidology.org)

CHAPTER FIFTEEN

Conclusion

I am now back at home and on different medication that should help me through this period of my life. I am so fed up of being scared all the time, I may just have to do something radical. No, not suicide, but I was thinking of facing my fear square on and see what happens. The best place for this is somewhere where I have no one but me to deal with. Maybe the Australian dessert...

Expression through my paintings

Below are the paintings I did over time as aids to express how I felt and to help me through bad attacks of depression

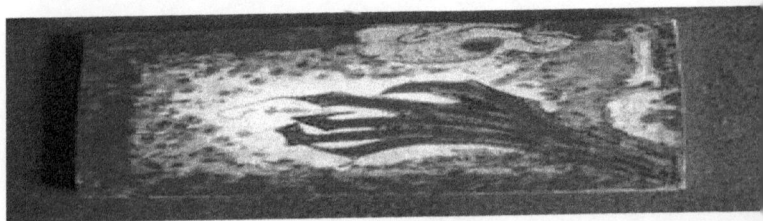

I wanted visualise the precursor to the depression. It is like the heavy knot in your solar plexus. With me it feels like a grizzly bony claw like hand that rips into my chest and try's to rip out my heart. This is what comes up from behind and side swipes me into the grip of depression. This is what I imagine the suppression and icy fear looks like. It pulls me down to the deep depths beyond the waves where I can't breath or see beyond the murky waters.

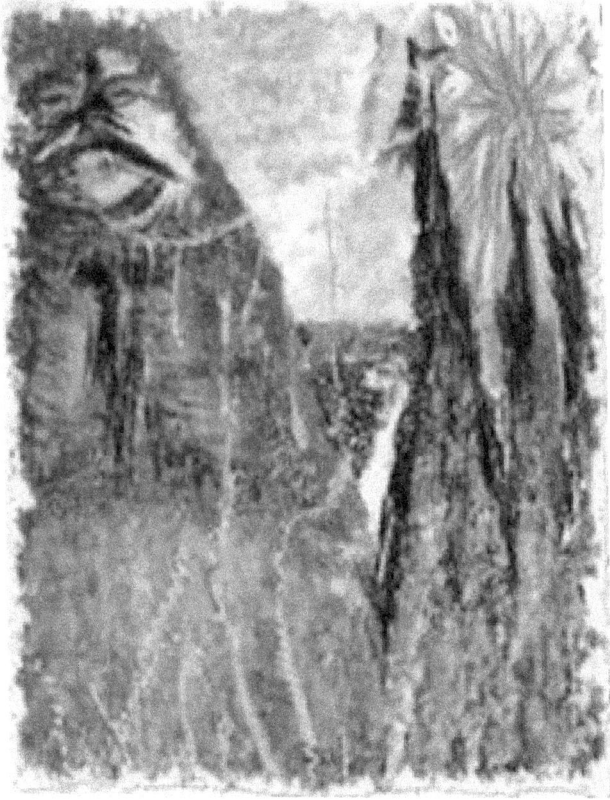

This picture is of the demon itself. I visualized what it would look like if it could be put into a form of some kind, with all the repressible nacasistic controlling qualities it holds in high stead... Therefore, I thought Jabba the Hut from Star Wars because he is hideously ugly and a parasite, which suits my image of this depression. I am on the pinnacle to the right with slime sticking to me from Jabber's mouth so as not to let me escape to freedom.

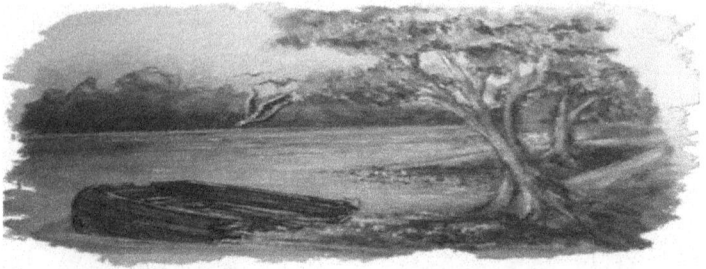

I painted this picture because I wanted to be away somewhere alone so as I couldn't go away on my own for a while this was what I did. It is of a boat that took me to a secret island. It fell apart in the effort to get me there where I was safe from the black thoughts...The drawing came out quite somber-looking but this was the best I could do with the way I felt. (No rainbows, no sunny days, too far up the ladder of optimism for me to visualize.) At the time of painting the picture, it was sheer effort for me to put brush to canvas. But I knew it would help stop the escalation of feeling desperate. I looked at the picture and it enabled me to be free. I was starting to come back to normality again. If it works, do it.

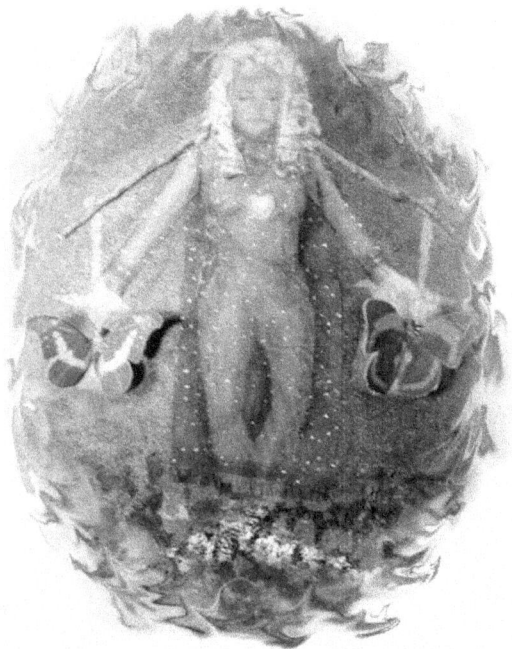

This picture has significant meaning for me. When my eldest son took charge of me from the psychiatric hospital, he took me to his house and sat me down, and in that quiet calming voice of his, requested I paint a specific scene. He has never done that before. (I have painted for years as therapy for myself.) His request was for me to understand and visualize the seriousness of giving up and the consequences of my actions. Also what it would do to him and his brother if I gave into this illness. So I thought about what he said. This is what I came up with. In the picture, I am trying to stay standing in a pit of burning coals. The white-hot coals represent the depression. This is hell and the only thing keeping me from crashing and burning are my children. The butterflies on each side of me symbolize my two sons. Butterflies have delicate wings and can be damaged very easily if touched. The heat has some effect on the wings but not enough to stop them flying, but there is some scorch marks on their body. At all costs, they must not get burned by the fires of hell (depression) and it is up to me to hold on and keep them safe, so I have.

The Invisible Stalker

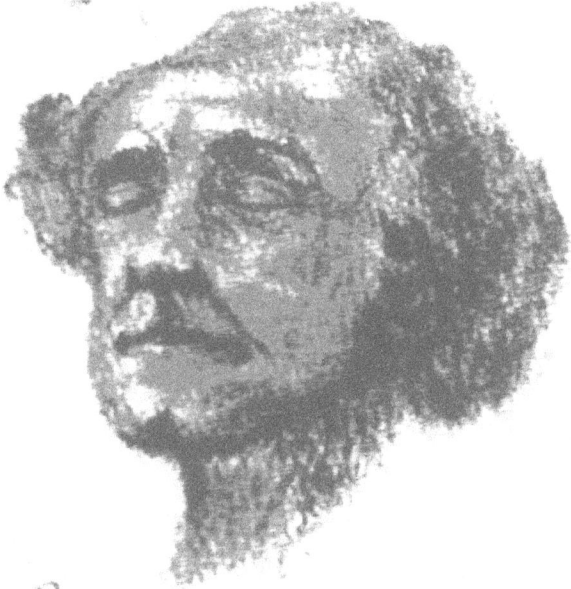

It may seem strange, but I painted this picture because I wanted to visualize a person who cared about me. A guardian, if you like, as there was no one in my life (parents). I ached for someone to care about me so this picture is my fantasy "father." I did not paint any eyes because I wanted him to be all knowing without having to see. It helped. I looked at this face and thought it was a kind face and had a wealth of love to give. I guess this is what young people are like when they have their imaginary friends. I put mine on canvas. Even now, twenty-two years later, I still think he is a kind man, and out there somewhere are kind people too who care. I guess I have a desperate need to be loved by a parent figure. (And I am now middle-aged and still feel like a lost child!) We all need to be loved no matter what our age.

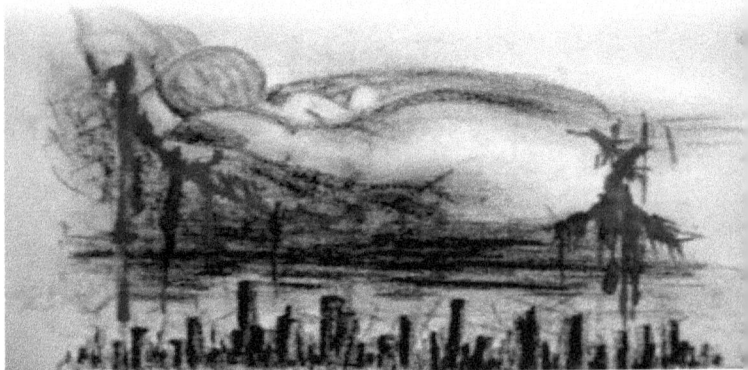

When I was younger and feeling alone and vulnerable, I always imagine being curled up in Jesus' hand (this was when I had faith, but cynicism has taken over since). But I still use this image when I feel vulnerable. The blood represented Jesus' sacrifice for me, but due to my lost faith, it now represents a "being," a "guardian angel" protecting me no matter how they hurt, as I would protect my sons against the ills of the world too. Can you see the irony in this last paragraph? I try to die, but I have this strong protectiveness towards my sons. The mind and its aberrations can cause such chaos in people's lives.

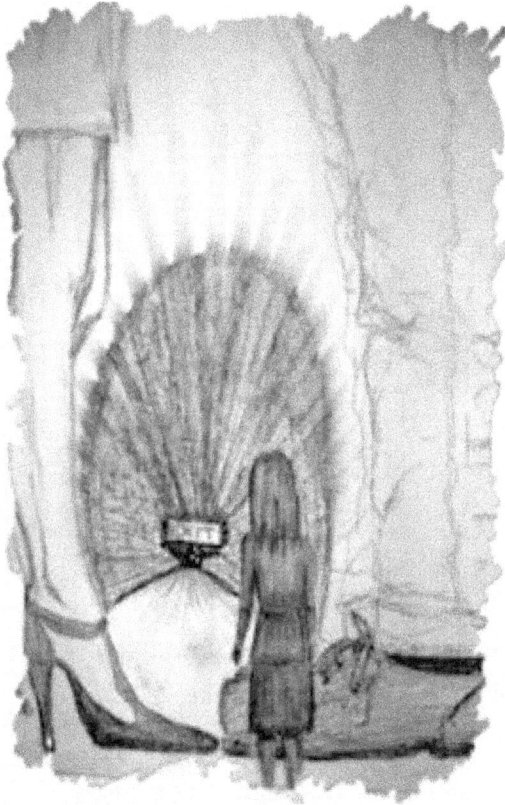

Quite often, a sense of worthlessness washes over me. This painting shows how I feel about me and the surrounding environment I am in at the time. People around me look so capable and confident. It only makes me feel worse. I am getting smaller and smaller. I feel so lost, not sure where I fit in. I felt I had nothing to contribute to life, no value. I always felt so insignificant and a waste of time to people.

Patricia Reid

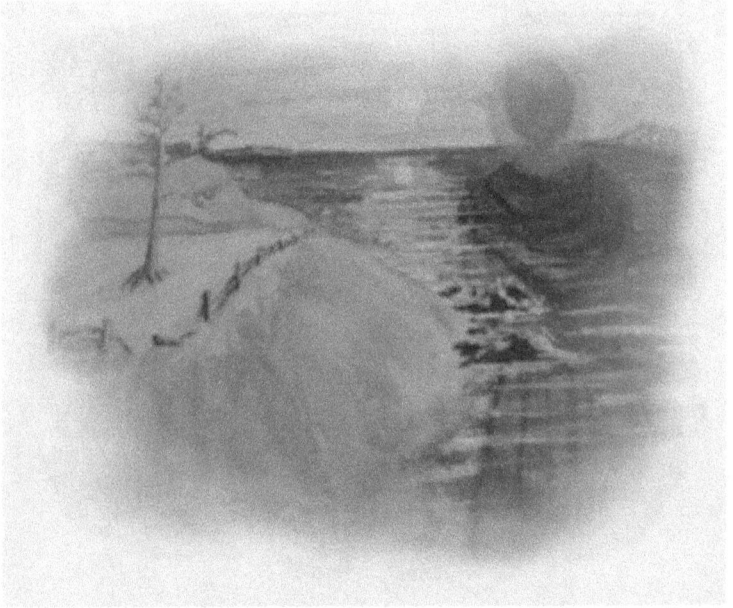

I sometimes feel invisible; like a non-entity. I felt this way since early adulthood. It is still just as strong as it was all those years ago. I am displaced; I don't seem to belong anywhere. To feel unwanted whether real or imagined is a lonely place.

The Invisible Stalker

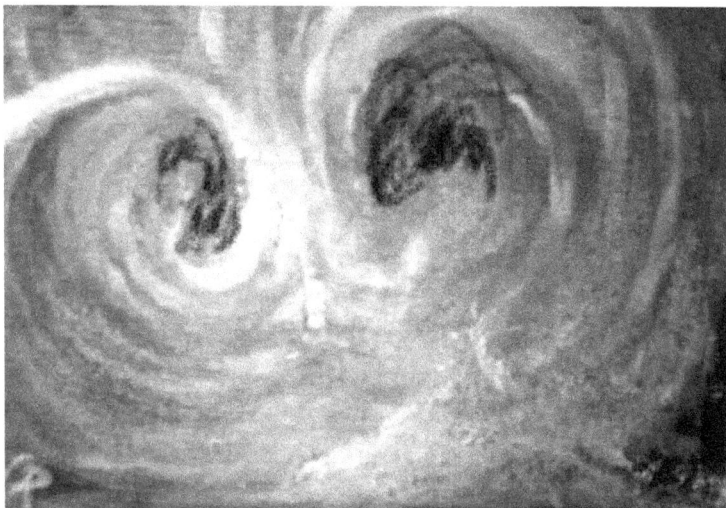

I painted this picture to try to comprehend what the hold on my mind, i.e. depression, looked like if I could see it. These massive waves crashing in on themselves represent the finality of it all. The depression is going on forever. I am in there somewhere and that is how it feels sometimes when I am having a really bad time of it. This represents the negative side of me, bashing me up and making pulp out of me and it doesn't stop... The power is too strong to fight. THAT is what it is like at the end, when you have no fight left in you.

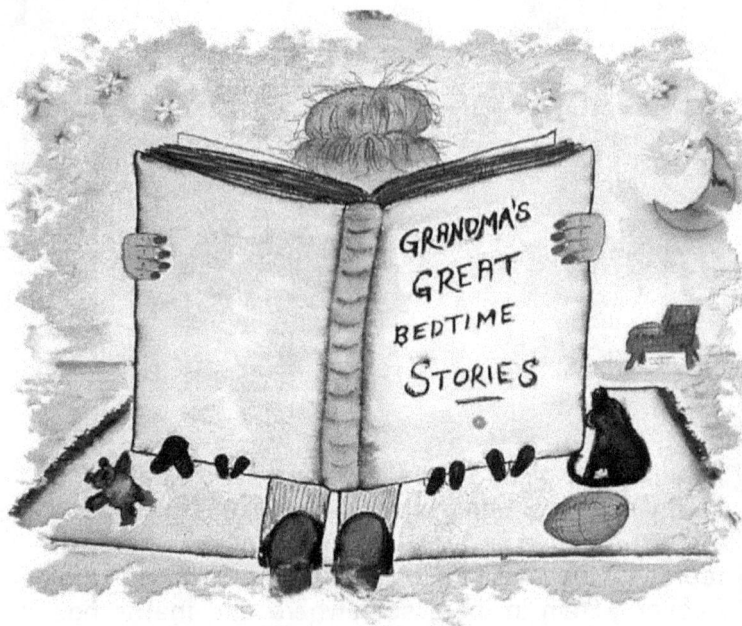

This is my latest painting, done in 2008. I dream of becoming a Grandma. I still have a lot of love to give. Most important, for the first time in my life I am looking to the future...Yeah, that's a good thing!

www.ingramcontent.com/pod-product-compliance
Lightning Source LLC
Chambersburg PA
CBHW031210270326
41931CB00006B/505